It's a Beautiful Day *for*

BOOT CAMP

Empowering cancer survivors with physical and mental toughness

by

Anita Kellman

with

Stewart Smith,
former USN (SEAL)

The It's a Beautiful Day for Boot Camp Workout e-book is sold on the following sites:
www.beatcancerbootcamp.com
www.stewsmith.com
www.military.com
www.policelink.com

And the published version paperback book can be found at local book retailers as well as
www.beatcancerbootcamp.com
www.stewsmith.com
www.amazon.com
www.bn.com

Contact the authors Anita Kellman and Stew Smith.
As part of the purchase, you do have access to email us at anytime and we will answer
your questions as soon as possible.
Below are the different ways to contact us:
www.Beatcancerbootcamp.com
and
www.stewsmith.com

Waiver of Liability

What you are about to undertake is an advanced fitness program. Injuries may occur in any workout program as with this specific program written by Anita Kellman and Stew Smith. By performing the program, you are waiving any liability to Anita Kellman or Stew Smith. This is a recommended program that has worked for many others. It may not be right for you. It is recommended that you consult a physician before undertaking any new fitness regimen.

ISBN 978-0-578-08019-2

"It's a Beautiful Day for Boot Camp" is dedicated to all my troop members who recognize, that each and every day is a beautiful day!

For Strength. For Health. For Life.

- "Sarge"

Acknowledgments

There are so many people I would like to acknowledge in helping me not only complete this book, but believed in my dream of reaching out to help others. I am very fortunate to have so many believers; it was impossible not to succeed.

First, I would like to thank my family, who have been so supportive over the years. I know it wasn't easy on them, having me always working on endless projects. Without their understanding, I wouldn't have had the opportunity to pursue my goals.

To Suzanne, who believed in my vision, and was right by my side to help me every step of the way. She gave me the strength to never give up. I am one of the lucky ones, not only to have such a good friend, but a true visionary as well.

To Nancy, who spent countless hours helping me put the story together and for reading this story again and again, and for enduring my minor crisis of confidence (and a couple of major ones). I know I couldn't have completed this book without her help. Her dedication and friendship is one I will always be grateful for.

To Adam, who jumped in, no questions asked and always helped with every project I needed. You have proved over and over again that there are caring people in the world willing to lend a hand.

To Kathleen, for bringing your nutrition expertise to this book, and writing the comprehensive and witty "Boot Camp Mess Hall."

To John, who pushed me to tell my story and forced me to find the writer within.

To my boot camp troops who shared their stories and are the heart and soul of this book.

And finally, to Stew, whose Navy SEAL fitness program became the foundation of Beat Cancer Boot Camp. Thank you for your generous offer to work on this book and get it published. I am truly touched by your commitment to help me not only with this book, but with my program. As you have said, "once you conquer doubt, you can do anything you put your mind to." Thank you for teaching me how to conquer doubt. Your words and encouragement throughout made this book possible.

Table of Contents

Foreword

The purpose of this book is to share with you the heartfelt stories along with the philosophy of Beat Cancer Boot Camp. This is much more than an exercise program — it's life changing for many. Although the exercise component is the basis of this program, it has evolved into much more.

I started this program over five years ago, with nothing more than a copy of *The Complete Guide to Navy SEAL Fitness*, by Stewart Smith. Years of fitness training, working with cancer patients and a whole lot of love and determination to help others came in handy, too. Using Stewart's book as my "bible," I created the Boot Camp program, even quoting some of his best motivational lines! The discipline and toughness fighting cancer is no different than that of Navy Seals training. Remain focused on your goals, not letting anything stop you.

I contacted Stewart a while back and asked if he did speaking engagements. I thought it would be so great to have him come out and speak. After all, his book inspired me, to reach out and inspire others. Talk about paying it forward. To my surprise, not only did he offer to come out, but wanted to get involved and help my program. This led to working together on other projects. I am thankful for his encouragement to continue with this book and to share my story with others.

Anita "Sarge" Kellman

Quite simply, Anita has given my written workout program much more meaning than I ever intended. Not only is my program helping young men and women train for the Naval Special Warfare / Operations Physical Screening Tests / Training, but NOW, through Anita Kellman, it is providing a health and fitness guide for cancer fighters. Thank you Anita, you made my book a lot more special.

I would also like to honor my mother Rae Smith and sister Liz Smith Pittinger who both have battled cancer bravely. A special and very personal love goes into writing this book for me and I am honored to be a part of such a worthy mission.

Stew Smith CSCS
former Navy SEAL

Introduction – What is Beat Cancer Boot Camp?

AN ATHLETE'S PERSPECTIVE:
By Bernard Lagat, *Olympic medalist and World Champion runner*

As a professional runner, I value my fitness more than the average person. To be the best in the world, I train tough daily, with the goal of being number one. When I was invited by Anita Kellman to attend one of her Boot Camp Classes, I knew it would be easy for me. After all, I am a professional athlete, and these Boot Camp members are recreational people, recovering from cancer.

I knew it was a group of cancer survivors. I thought it was a neat idea, and I would go in there, teach them a few simple exercises, and give them some motivation to work out. I thought the troop members would be physically weak, depressed, and quite honestly, a group that needed cheering up. After all, they were all dealt a pretty crappy set of cards!

But wow, I was in for a surprise. These guys are dressed in Boot Camp gear, and Anita was yelling at them! They were full of energy, jumping up and down, running around, hanging off bars, doing push-ups, — now that I recall, I think EVERYBODY was yelling! I just stood there in awe. The group was making jokes, laughing, encouraging each other, all while Anita bossed them around!

I remember seeing a lady with no hair, another doing modified exercises because she is recovering from a mastectomy, and a husband tearing up … yes, the man was the one with tears!

He was crying because he couldn't believe how happy his wife was, and he was so grateful that his wife has this support group that is giving her the energy and will to fight cancer. After seeing him, I almost teared up myself. But Anita didn't give me the time or chance. She yelled at me to drop and give her 10 … I just did as told. Then I had to do another 10, and another 10, and then run to the next station, and do curl ups. Another 10! Another 10! Another 10!

Yes, I am a professional runner, Olympic silver medalist, World Champion, second fastest 1500 meter runner of all time, and I had to admit, I couldn't keep up with the troop. They ended up gathering around me, yelling at me. (OK, they were encouraging me, but I was so embarrassed, it felt like they were yelling!) It was mostly cheering and, of course, counting. I was in pain, and they were having fun.

I admire everything about Beat Cancer Boot Camp, their organization, their commitment, and their support. I give them the utmost respect. They are a bunch of "Lance Armstrongs" in Boot Camp gear! They have taught me a lot about life, and my own goals. I exercise as part of my profession, with the goal to be number one. They work out to survive, it's a battle for the rest of their lives – and we all only have one.

A POLICE OFFICER'S VIEW:

By Richard Harper, Captain, Tucson Police Department, Retired

I can remember my first encounter with Anita Kellman a few years ago. I was a middle-aged police commander, trying to maintain my fitness level, and spend quality time with my wife, going through "Basic Training Workouts" as part of a City of Tucson sponsored fitness program. It was a small class, but the people involved were all motivated to be more fit. I noticed that Anita did not come to play but to train.

One day we were doing 50-yard wind sprints. Now Anita might be all of 5 feet tall, so you know she was running at least 3 strides for every one of mine, and she was matching me yard for yard. As we neared the finish line, I desperately lunged, and if I hadn't she would have clearly beaten me. I was a spent police hero, but I hadn't lost, even though I walked through the rest of the workouts. I got a quick wink from Anita that day, and she said, "Nice workout. Hoorah." I know now that she had to have slowed down to let me save face.

I saw Anita again a few years later at a Breast Cancer walk, and she was adorned in a fashionable camouflaged outfit leading a group of women at the city's central park. Now these women were not just walking, but every few minutes they would stop their cadence and get down and do 25 push-ups before moving on. It took me right back to my Army basic training days at Fort Jackson, South Carolina. And out front leading was "Sarge," Anita Kellman.

I attended their workout at Brandi Fenton Park, and arrived toward the end of the session. There was Anita, down in the front leaning rest position and counting out pushups while the twenty or so women worked to keep pace. This was the beginning of summer, and in Tucson the summers are not just hot they are brutally hot. The women were on pushup number 50, as I recall, and continued for another 10. But I think Anita did maybe twenty more pushups.

My plan was to "educate" these nice women about the Tucson Police Foundation and our community event, but it was really me who received an education I will never forget. You see, Cancer treatments and their side effects can dramatically alter a person's appearance. There were women there without hair, without breasts, some having gained some weight due to cancer fighting drugs as well as the emotional impact that all of these physical changes can have on an individual.

Each woman introduced herself to me and then told me a short story about her encounter with cancer. I was amazed at the inner strength that these women had and with their hilarious sense of humor! It did get a little raunchy, and I had to threaten to take out my handcuffs. Of course, I had so many volunteers, we all laughed until we couldn't breathe.

As each woman spoke, she talked about the importance of the fitness program and the support that they all gave each other. But the common theme that came out was how important Anita's program was, how her leadership had such a positive impact on their lives. Anita gave them back the power of control over their lives, to build their self esteem through fitness. She gave them an attitude of can-do, and of friendship, not just superficial, but a deep long-lasting, unconditional love that helps a person get through those "tough moments."

I walked away after the meeting a changed man. With over 34 years as a cop, I have experienced a few life-changing events. I had a deep profound respect for all of these women, fighting the good fight, diligently working out each week to get control of their own lives and to share their joys and fears with their Boot Camp group. And I realized what an important person that "Sarge" Anita Kellman was to the lives of each and every one of these individuals.

THE SURVIVOR'S PERSPECTIVE:
By Michael Blake, Author, *Dances With Wolves*

Physical downturns, including large ones, are a part of life on this planet.

To be struck with cancer is devastating but is only the beginning. Surviving the treatment, maintaining a positive look at the future and making vows to use the time you earn … all are difficult to achieve. Taking a new look at maintaining a body that was struck is a move that can help achieve a return to the beauty of life. Ironically, having cancer can give those afflicted opportunities to move forward in ways that are rare.

The story of Beat Cancer Boot Camp is one that provides an opportunity for all to look beyond the disease, to clench their fists and make a fight for more life with mental power that few humans have.

About the Authors

Anita Kellman

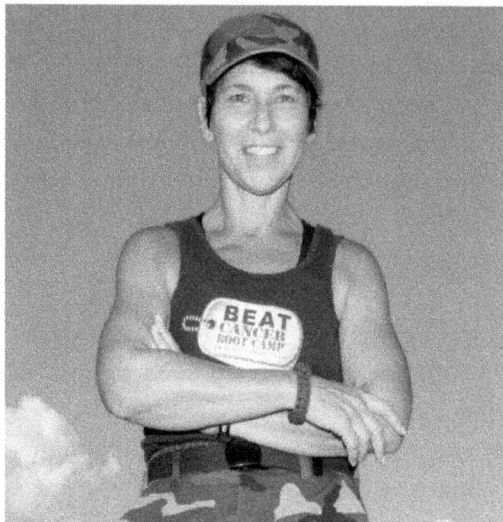

Kellman has worked in the medical field for over 25 years and is a clinical liaison for patients undergoing biopsies and other procedures. Through her work, she meets cancer survivors every day — in various stages of treatment and recovery — and most of them are looking for a way to cope more effectively. Beginning in 2001, Kellman attended Boot Camp classes and learned Navy Seal exercises, and in 2004 she adapted these techniques to start an intensive support group built around physical fitness instead of "woe is me". Kellman shares her knowledge, experience, and infectious enthusiasm. She is recognized throughout the Tucson community for her contribution to cancer awareness, and women's health.

Visit the Official Website:
www.beatcancerbootcamp.com

About the Authors

Stew Smith CSCS

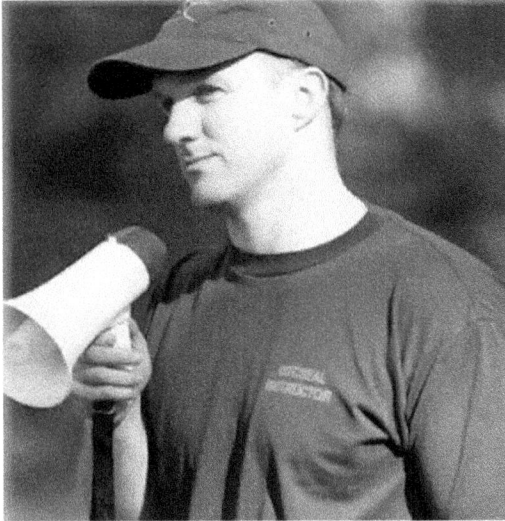

Stew Smith is a graduate of the U.S. Naval Academy, a former Navy SEAL, and author of several fitness and self defense books such as *The Complete Guide to Navy SEAL Fitness, Maximum Fitness*, and *SWAT Fitness*.

Certified by the National Strength and Conditioning Association as a Strength and Conditioning Specialist (CSCS) and as military fitness trainer, Smith trains students for Navy SEAL, Special Forces, SWAT, FBI, ERT and many other law enforcement professions.

Little did he know his products would also be a part of a much more meaningful program than scoring higher on fitness tests. Through Kellman and the Beat Cancer Boot Camp program, workouts by Stew Smith have an even greater importance — helping people fight cancer.

His articles and books at StewSmith.com, Military.com, NavySEALs.com and PoliceLink.com can help you achieve your fitness goals, whether you're a beginner or advanced.

Contact Stew Smith at **StewSmith.com** for any answers to your fitness questions.

"You gain strength, courage, and confidence by every experience in which you really stop to look fear in the face. You must do the thing which you think you cannot do."

– Eleanor Roosevelt

Chapter One: It's a Beautiful Day for Boot Camp!

I bend over and lace up my combat boots. They're filthy. Dust on the top, mud caked on the bottom. They are definitely worn out after all these years. I meticulously tuck my fatigues into my boots before I tie them. I put on my Boot Camp shirt and make sure I have my whistle with me. I'm ready. No matter the weather or my mood, it's always a beautiful day for Boot Camp. I don't care if it's 30° or 105°, raining or unbearably hot, Boot Camp always happens, and I always wear the same outfit.

I arrive at the park one hour before revelry. It's empty and quiet. I unlock the Beat Cancer Boot Camp Headquarters, an old house converted into a park's office. Through some strategic planning (and successful pleading), I acquired this space three years ago. The troops gathered, and we had a painting party to clean, decorate and make it our own. I made sure the walls were painted an appropriate color: khaki. After all we are Boot Camp! We even have our very own camo-decorated bathroom. I'm so proud.

A few early birds start arriving. We chat about anything and everything. They look at me and ask, "What do we need today?" Translation: they want to know what plans I have up my sleeve for class. It doesn't matter what I tell them they need, they always whine and moan about it. We start to set up snacks for after class, which is as important to most as the workout itself.

It's time to go outside and mingle with everyone. I love just being there and listening to them share what's going on. We are a very tight knit group and many of the women have been involved since the group began five years ago. I've seen relationships evolve from acquaintances going to an exercise class to lifelong friends. It never ceases to amaze me that they are so enthusiastic about this class. I finally realized it is more about the people than the exercise. Whatever works.

Out comes my whistle and I let it rip. "Attention!!!" Class is about to begin. They all start slowly getting into the warm up position. I'm always overwhelmed when I look at these incredible people. Sometimes it's hard for me to focus. I've met many of these women through the doctor's office where I work. I've performed their biopsies. I know their diagnosis. I know their fears, and I strive to give them hope. I blow the whistle again, which helps me stay focused. "It's a beautiful day for Boot Camp!" I shout. A few regulars roll their eyes, and I prepare for the start of our marching cadence.

I remember the day I came up with the cadence. I was training for a half marathon, and running on this terrible, hilly eight-mile loop in the desert. It was a hot day, and

I was running on this road alone with nothing but my thoughts. I was engrossed in trying to keep my mind occupied at the time, so I would finish this run. The only thing that would keep me focused was thinking about Boot Camp. I started babbling all different cadences. There wasn't anyone around to hear me, so I chanted all the variations until I came up with the one I liked. Yes, this one was perfect. It said it all.

"I don't know what you've been told. We are brave and we are bold. We will do more than survive. We are strong and we will thrive! Sound off... 1, 2. Sound off... 3, 4. Sound off 1, 2, 3, 4... 1, 2!"

Rain or shine, hot or cold, class always starts the same. It's consistent. I do believe there would be an uproar if I altered that part of the routine. With the ever-changing landscape of their health, there's comfort in having something they can depend on.

In the next hour we move from stretches, to weights, to cardio, to massive amounts of push-ups... all with much laughter and complaining. They fall back into their groups. It's kind of like Junior High with all the cliques but without the 13 year old hormones. The group consists of haves and have-nots, professionals and housewives, grandmothers and college students. Cancer doesn't discriminate. It is an equalizer. I've seen that common bond break through the typical social barriers.

Out to the field we go to begin our lower body routine. I try to line them up for this, but it's always a challenge. Yak, yak, yak… I notice a troop member constantly talking.

In my best Sarge voice I say, "We are not working on our jaw muscles. We are working our quads!" Arlene smiles and gingerly replies, "My jaw is in great shape, and, by the way, I can multi-task." Now I'll be tough, throw in some cardio. That usually shakes them up, and hopefully keeps them quiet! Here comes the moaning and groaning.

"What are we doing?" Another Boot Camp member whines. "Are you NOT paying attention for a change?" I sarcastically ask.

I seem to expect this from her on a routine basis, often a couple times during class. After five years of taking this class, she enjoys me getting in her face, almost as much as I like dishing it out. It is our ritual – something constant. It is one of those things that just does not change.

Onward we go to the Circle of Doom, as they lovingly call it. We head back to the grassy area to complete the session. You see, some clever Boot Camp member came up with that name because the area is shaped in a circle. The last part of class is always pushups and ab work, hence the name... Circle of Doom.

I yell back at them, "I always thought it was the circle of love!"

Knowing that we do at least one hundred pushups now, they give me hard time about it. I give it right back. They expect it, and probably look forward to it. Well ... maybe not, but I always remind them they've earned bragging rights when they're done. Come on now, how many people can say they do over a hundred pushups? Getting ready to do the last stretch, they all give out a loud scream. Who hoo!! It's over. Again, another ritual they all seem to enjoy.

Someone is asking about the snacks? Who brought snacks? Are they ready? Should they go into the building to start the coffee? I learned a long time ago, it is best if I come early and prepare the kitchen, than to have them all fight about who should help set up! After any announcements of what's coming up with Boot Camp, they collect their belongings and head back to the kitchen.

This is where some of the best informal mentoring takes place. We all hang around there for around one hour, eating, drinking, laughing and sharing stories. Some purely personal things, some related to cancer issues. It all depends on who is there that day, and especially if anyone is new to the group. The newbies always get an earful. I do remind them – what happens at Boot Camp, stays at Boot Camp!

This is one of the safest environments they could be in. No one judges you on your looks, fears, or insecurities. There isn't someone who hasn't gone through just about anything that would be asked. I laugh as I hear some stories from "girls night out" that some of them attended. Nothing I hear fazes me anymore. From their sexual experiences, to their sexual preferences, there is nothing they don't share.

It does amaze me, to see this group so close with each other, and coming from such diverse backgrounds. The truth is many of our paths would have not crossed if they didn't have the common denominator of cancer. Sometimes I feel in a fog, understanding how important this is to everyone, and wondering how I could keep this going. Keep them going. This is the lifeline to so many. Boot Camp is such a difference maker, and to see how some of them have enhanced, not only their appearance throughout this, but also their lives. I put on my "Sarge" face and realize this must continue, and I have to reach out to more recruits.

Looking around I see a troop member I met when performing her biopsy. When I told her about Boot Camp, she insisted that she is not a support group person.

Thanks but no thanks. After all she is young, and newly married, and perhaps by avoiding a group like this she feels she is not affected by cancer. I encouraged her to at least come to a dinner and meet some of these women. There are many who are young that she can relate too. After all, it would be good for her to see the troops laughing, smiling, and most importantly, alive and thriving.

She did come, and even tried a class. She was hooked. She continued coming throughout her chemo treatments, and today is the first day she came to class with no hat on – just a few scruffy hairs coming in on her head. She stood tall, and was confident with herself. This made me cry. I have to look away, as not to get emotional in front of the group today. After all, I am the "Sarge" and they expect me to be tough and push them beyond their limits. It's tough love. Another success story from this program, and it changed her life, and so many others, in so many ways. This is what keeps me going.

I make sure the building is all cleaned up and lock the doors. I have to hurry home now to clean up, and go into work. I usually don't work on Boot Camp days, but I was asked to help out today. Taking a shower, and changing into my work clothes, I leave Sarge behind for now.

I work in a breast surgeon's office. I understand everyone who comes here is frightened. I try to put them at ease, as I bring them back to the room to meet the doctor. Being his clinical liaison, I am there for the patient. We have a new patient who is pretty young, in her 30's. There is something abnormal on her mammogram, so I explain to her that we will be doing a biopsy. As I'm setting up the room, and explaining the procedure to her, I couldn't help but think, she would fit in with the Boot Camp group.

I try not to solicit every person who enters my office, but there are some that I know would benefit from this program. It is always a very delicate situation and I'm careful when I mention this to them. Making small talk first with her, I contemplate if this would be a good time. We have a monthly dinner, and it happens to be tonight. Hmmm. I think about it for a while. What the hell? I blurt out all about Boot Camp and to my surprise she knew all about it already. I told her it's her lucky day, and she could come as my guest to our monthly dinner tonight. She took my card, and said she'd call me later.

Three more biopsies until I take my lunch break. I can't wait because I usually try to do some Boot Camp business over my lunch. Sarge is back. There are always follow up calls to be made. I want to check in with some of the members who recently had surgery. I am concerned about a few of them, and don't feel an email would be appropriate. Of course, I am not the nice touchy-feely type of person, even when I call. I usually start off by telling them that they can't use surgery as an excuse to not exercise. Neither is chemo! They know better than to feel sorry for themselves. I just won't let them. I push them verbally as much as physically. They love it.

My break is almost over and I have to return to the office and, again, leave Sarge behind. It is time for me to be the caring compassionate person. It gets so difficult to always be changing roles. There are times I get mixed up and forget who I am. The sarcasm rolls off my tongue. This is great for Boot Camp, but not so great in a doctor's office.

I look at my watch and start to panic. It is 4:00, and I have to once again change clothes to become Sarge. I have to confess, I feel most comfortable dressed as Sarge. I use to think that was my alter ego, now I think that's me. I am Sarge. I quickly make some calls between patients, to make sure, everything is all set for the dinner. There are so many details to be taken care of. Tonight we are expecting 36 women, with a few newbies joining us. Oh yeah, I have to call that new girl from this morning and see if she's coming tonight.

Rushing back to the Boot Camp office, I make sure the tables are set up properly, and we are ready to go. Tonight we are having a guest speaker, so I want to make sure everything is running on time. I am getting tired, because it's been a long day, but I quickly get some energy when the troops start arriving. This monthly dinner means so much to them. This is a great time for the informal mentoring to take place.

Once everyone is seated with their food, we go around and give a brief introduction. I keep looking at my watch, making sure we are on schedule for the speaker. Tonight we are learning about nutrition. I have to give a quick disclaimer, since we are having pizza, pasta, and birthday cake. Oh I did throw in a healthy salad, too!

I was pleased so many people came, and some new members exchanged numbers. This is how it all starts with Boot Camp. I look around the room and see them laughing and joking with each other. Some look like they are in a deep conversation. Some are there to just get their "fix" of each other. I am always astonished to see how close these women have become. Though I feel some emotion coming on, I must remain strong in front of them. I take out my whistle and blow it loudly. It is time for announcements. I am in Sarge mode once again.

It's time to clean up from the dinner and finally head home for the evening. I'm wiped out and looking forward to a good night's sleep because tomorrow will be just as busy. At ease!

Chapter Two: Your Mother Wears Combat Boots

I thought of so many things to say about my mom. Something that would say how amazing she is, or how I know that she helps so many people. In addition to all the other million of things there are to say about my mom, a simple three words come into mind, "I love you. " She has inspired me to take on challenges in school and … well … just overall life. I could not have thanked her enough. My mom has managed working a stressful job, putting this book together, Boot Camp, and just being my mom.

I have put her down — not meaning to — about how she is too busy and not there for me. In reality, my mom is always there for me, and then I realized I had to be there for her. I started going to Boot Camp and just like that I met many amazing women who shared their story with me and really made me look up to them.

I soon realized what my mom was doing and then understood why this group meant so much to her. After that day I became closer with my mom. I felt like I connected to her. Boot camp was soon something I loved to be involved in. There were the outdoors, the people, and their lives. It was just magic. That's maybe the word …magic. Boot Camp brings a different story, and helps out people in so many ways, and simply, I am grateful for that. I love my mom.

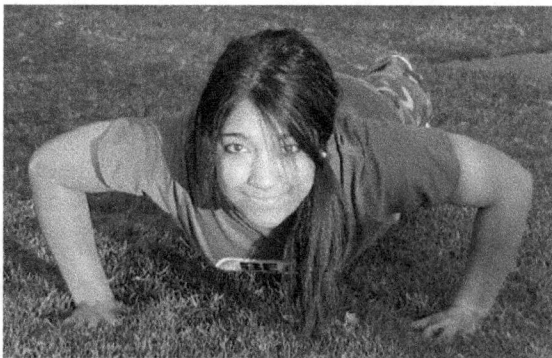

Marlee Kellman

The Beginning

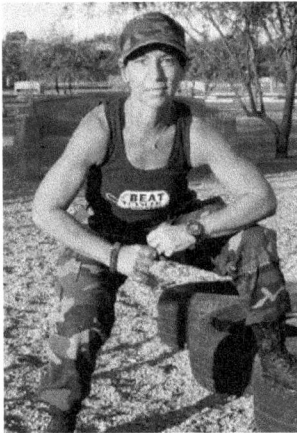

Five years ago … while taking Advil in the morning to relieve some of the swelling and pain in my elbows, I wondered, "What did I do?"

Oh, right. Two days ago, I was in the park, completing my "super set" of pull-ups. I had enlisted in a weekend warrior exercise class through the City, and was determined not to stop short of the set. There were only a few women attending this class. Needless to say, we were all quite competitive, and not one of us, was willing to give up. So, foolishly, we all suffered the consequences of our egos.

We called each other and laughed about it, how we all looked like Popeye with swollen arms. We wore it like a badge of honor, proving to ourselves, that we were not only determined, but also strong in our own right. I couldn't wait for the next class, to see what other challenges lay ahead. My mission was to push myself beyond my expectations. So began my love affair, with all things, Boot Camp.

Actually my story starts years before a class in Tucson. I'm Chicago-born and raised and the middle child and only girl in a tight-knit working class family. My childhood memories mostly consist of the time growing up in
Albany Park. My parents, along with my Aunt and Uncle, owned a duplex. My aunt, uncle and three cousins (two girls and a boy) lived on the first floor, while we had the second floor. The only doors that were kept locked were the main doors to the building. The landing between the two floors was our play area, equipped with all our toys. Since we were all around the same age, the basement was a giant adventure for us as well. Although we kept separate households, we were very much like a community. The need to reach out to others was not a priority to me, because I was always surrounded by my family.

There was a neighborhood girl, though, who I did meet when we were around 8 years old. We became friends. It was convenient because she lived just down the block on the other side of the alley.

I was always small. My new friend was much bigger than me. It never bothered me, but I found out it bothered her. So to make her feel better about herself, at the age of ten, we started a secret club. Only the two of us were members. We called it Healthy Girls, but it was our secret. Careful not to be exposed for what we were doing, we gave it a code name, HG. Our slogan was "HG we will be!"

Little did I know, my passion for helping others probably began right then. In our HG Club, I made a chart of exercises that we had to complete each day. They were pretty much all the old standard exercises, jumping jacks, toe touches and arm circles. (Ha! Kind of what I do now in my Boot Camp classes. Who knew?) The part that made it successful was we had a focus, and were working towards a goal. It was something to last a lifetime and not a quick fix.

You see, part of my initial motivation was watching my Mom always struggle on diets. I knew all along, I would never want to live my life like that, and even told her so. It just seemed so much easier to adapt a healthier way to live. I enjoyed watching my friend, knowing she was doing something positive for herself.

As I got a little older, I was trying to figure out what I wanted to do when I grew up. When I was 15, I took a volunteer job as a candy striper. I couldn't think of a better way than to get the experience of working in a hospital. I quickly figured out that being a nurse or working in a lab was not for me. I liked the patient contact, but wanted a broader, quicker way to meet patients. The idea of Radiographer was a perfect fit for me!

At the age of 18, I was accepted into the best hospital-based program in Chicago, Michael Reese Hospital. It was an intense 24-month program. I was required to live in the nurse's residence, and had no summer breaks. The school accepted 12 people in the program each year. It was difficult but exciting to be part of that program.

There were so many breakthroughs happening at that time with x-ray. Some of my friends at school decided to specialize in CAT scans, a new and upcoming field. I on the other hand, chose mammography. That was also brand new. There weren't even dedicated mammography machines yet; they were using x-ray machines and experimenting with Xerox mammography. Mammography and women's health in general were an up-and-coming field. I just felt it.

When I first moved to Tucson, I was newly married, and knew no one! I remembered my mother was always in groups, and that was very much her social life. Consequently, I quickly became involved in groups and met all kinds of interesting women. Being involved to me was not a passive role. I just don't understand anything passive. So, I slowly moved up the ranks of the organization, and didn't stop until I was the chapter president, which I took very seriously.

As my family grew, so did my lifestyle. I was working part-time, mainly to keep up in my field, and to do something outside the home that felt rewarding. As a mother

of four children, I was looking for a chance to do something for myself, and yes…
by myself. It gets tricky trying to find that time, without feeling guilty. I became
involved in my children's school, and the old patterns returned. I did not stop until I
was PTA president. It made me feel good to not only be doing something to help my
children, but to make a difference to others.

As time passed though, I felt it was time for a shift to get involved additional
endeavors. I joined a social action group, thinking this would be the right fit.
Helping people in need who appreciate my efforts was right up my alley.

To no one's surprise, I worked my way up to become Chairperson in this very large
and quite powerful community group. This diverse organization sponsored activities
that included national politicians, along with community and religious leaders.
I couldn't believe I was the one who led them for two years, even winning the
prestigious Paul Newman award for "Make a Difference Day."

After working so hard to make my contribution a success, I was passed over for an
esteemed "Woman of the Year" award. I was devastated when I realized how that
recognition was tied to a dollar amount. I donated the hours — not cash — because
there are better ways to make a difference than simply writing a check. I felt like
someone punched me in the stomach and knocked the wind out of me. I did not feel
validated for all I did. My bubble burst. And right or wrong, I walked away from the
organization.

The community of friends I met while volunteering allowed me to start weaving a
tapestry of diverse dynamic people. Little did I realize that this network would play
a significant role in the evolution of what would become my true passion — Beat
Cancer Boot Camp.

Trying to move forward, I fell back on something that was within my comfort zone
— exercise. I asked a friend who was taking a Boot Camp class at a local park if I
could join her. She was delighted to share this with me. It was not only a way for me
to take charge of my life, but to stay connected with friends.

During this time, a participant of the class was diagnosed with cancer. I was working
at a hospital at that time, and was well connected in the medical field of women's
health. I guided her through myriad doctor's appointments and surgeries. I was there
for her throughout her course of treatment. Our whole class was. We even bought
her a Navy Seals t-shirt to wear to her chemo treatments. We thought it would make
her feel tough. It did.

Realizing that exercise played an important role in recovery, we continued the classes and even encouraged others to join. It was difficult for the City to find an instructor to commit to the class for any length of time. I was asked to take over and teach the class. I gladly accepted the challenge. I liked teaching. I like motivating and helping others. What a perfect fit.

I met new patients who might be interested in an exercise program at the hospital. After doing biopsies on some women, I would get a good feel if they would be receptive. I knew this was not for everyone and I was selective on who I approached. The hospital was not supportive of my program, so that made it a bit tricky trying to solicit members.

I believed in the cause, so I really didn't care what the administration thought. I was always the patient advocate/rebel trying to watch out for them.
I left the hospital and started working for a breast surgeon who embraced my idea of an exercise program to uplift and renew cancer survivors. The first Boot Camp classes for cancer survivors only had six women. I took this role quite serious. I bought a book, *The Complete Guide to Navy SEAL Fitness* by Stewart Smith. I went to a military surplus store and purchased my first ever set of fatigues, and combat boots. Quite a change of dress from what I was use to. There was something magical when I dressed the part. I felt so empowered, so strong, and really tough. I couldn't wait to try it out the next day at class.

Standing in the front of the class, outdoors at the park, I yelled at them to stand in line. Roll call was about to begin, and it was by last name only. Just like the military. There was no cracking a smile on my part. At first I felt like I was in a play, just acting. It didn't take long for me to feel this was real, and I was comfortable doing this. We had our first workout, and I was so proud. Even more proud when I looked down at my boots, and saw the mud on them. This is Boot Camp after all, we should be getting dirty.

Fighting cancer is a battle, and I will take charge and help them get through this. I will show them there is nothing they can't do if they put their mind to it. There is nothing to stop them. I will guide them how to look fear in the face, and do the thing they thought they couldn't do. They will be strong. They will survive. Indeed they will thrive!

I found my calling.

Anita Kellman AKA "Sarge"

"We are all faced with a series of great opportunities brilliantly disguised as impossible situations."

- Charles R. Swindoll

Chapter Three: For Strength – Breaking Barriers

Becoming physically stronger

Interfacing with many newly diagnosed cancer survivors, I have noticed there seems to be a universal concern, "How am I ever going to get through this? Will I get through this? Where do I begin?"

You see, I understand their concerns, because I have seen this all before, and they have not. They didn't ask for this — it was thrown in their faces. They want to ask appropriate questions, but don't even know where to start. Their lives suddenly seem out of control. They are being pulled in different directions, going through the motions, but feeling totally out of control, with no choices. Do this. Go see this doctor. Do that. This is where the challenge begins. This is the time they must look fear in the face. The biggest fear — Will I survive?

To me this is a critical time to engage people into the program. It is important for them to know they are not alone. Others have gone through the same thing, and guess what, they are here today, and will be here tomorrow, laughing, joking around and sharing stories. Being surrounded by positive upbeat people who share your experiences is really helpful.

I love it when someone new hears about this group, and the first thing they tell me is, "I'm not a support group person."

I reply, "Perfect, you'll fit right in. This is not the touchy-feely support group you previously might have experienced. This is unique. We have a take-charge attitude that you might not be used to. But better start getting used to it! I will not allow you to feel sorry for yourself. There are no pity parties here."

It doesn't take much time to convince them they can do this, and they will. Ahhh … the power of positive thinking. Being a survivor starts with strength from within. You have to want it. I will make them feel it.

Welcome to Boot Camp. You've been drafted!

It is challenging to give survivors the strength they need at a time they feel so weak. Not physically weak, but emotionally. They feel disappointment that their bodies have failed them, and don't understand how because they don't feel sick. Well, let's get over all that and move on. There is no looking back, that doesn't serve a purpose. Let's show everyone the new face of cancer — one that is strong, determined, and not about to give up.

Research has shown that exercise helps in so many ways, including prevention of recurrence of cancer as well as prevention. Being physically stronger makes you mentally tougher. Mental toughness is a key factor in getting through the process.

First you have to break the mindset that having cancer means you're weak. You will quickly find out how tough you really are. It sometimes takes a challenge to overcome obstacles. Putting yourself through physical challenges will bring changes in your life you never thought could happen. Once you start taking charge of your physical health, everything else falls in place. It really does snowball.

You will not only feel stronger, but will be able to take control of your life. You will start seeing yourself in a whole new light. Being surrounded by positive people will empower you to new heights. Not only will it give you the strength to ask questions, it will help you to better understand your new life. It is just a new baseline and a different way to monitor and think about things. Not bad, just different. Just as your physical looks may change through all this, so will your attitude. Cancer picked the wrong person, and I'll prove it.

My co-author and inspiration Stew Smith can explain it better than I can.

Where does Mental Toughness come from? By Stew Smith

After I appeared on the National Geographic Channel's Fight Science television show about hypothermia and Special Ops, the emails I received discussed mental toughness as if I had some magic solution for people to acquire it. The truth is the human body is built for survival and will adapt to better handle cold, heat, stress, pain, and even illness. We are survival machines!

After years of training in cold water before, during and after my seven years in the SEAL Teams, I got used to colder water as seen in the Fight Science TV show. However, if you take a look at a definition of mental toughness, you will see that we all have something in life, sports, environment, or attitude that makes us a little bit tougher. If you do a search online on the subject, you will see a variety of mental toughness techniques, articles, stories of remarkable physical performances to brave acts of heroism overcoming insurmountable odds and fear. There are thousands of ways to get "mentally tough" and physical fitness is just one of many ways.

Mental Toughness has many definitions and is not limited to athletic performance and pain tolerance. I have known many men and women throughout my life who

I would define as "mentally tough." From an 85-year-old gardener to a high school wrestling friend, neither of whom ever had a bad day, much of mental toughness is simply attitude and self-esteem.

Personally, my philosophy has always been quite simple when it comes to mental toughness as well as increasing your body's ability to withstand pain. As I stated, my way is NOT the only way, just the catalyst I have used in the past to develop what I call mental and physical toughness that enabled me to graduate SEAL training more than fifteen years ago. It works for me and many others who have attended physically challenging events/training programs.

I believe that in athletics, especially that tough workouts will build mental toughness. Physiologically your body will start to buffer lactate (handle fatigue/pain) better, if you give it the stimulus to do so. Meaning we will physically adapt to get in better shape, and our muscles will fail later and later and later until you can surpass perceived limitations. In a military environment, this method has been known to work, BUT adding training under stress, hunger, and fatigue will only enhance performance on the battlefield. I guess the saying, "The more you bleed in training, the less you bleed in war," applies to this philosophy.

Mental Toughness requires tough conditioning, but there is a fine line between pain and injury, of course. This takes hundreds of reps of exercises (both physical and military ops), equivalent to non-stop punching for a boxer. In my case, enormously high reps of pushups, situps, pullups, dips, running for miles and swimming for miles will create increased energy levels, increased ability to buffer lactate, and an increased pain tolerance through training in the pain zone. **You really have to get the body to know what pain is before you can endure it longer.** Once again PAIN is not injury — but if you push too hard through pain you will be setting up for injury, so knowing your training limits is necessary as well.

And then the next day when you feel like crap, and you have to WILL yourself to workout again. THAT too is mental toughness. Persistence and determination are all factors as well. Other terms used to describe mental toughness are inspiration, self motivation and confidence.

In the end, to define such an intangible quality is almost impossible. There have been many people who do not exercise at all who bring themselves out of horrible childhoods of poverty, neglect, and illness to become heroes, mentors, millionaires, and presidents. That takes mental toughness in MY book, and they achieved it another way.

I have seen personally the struggle with cancer by my own mother, who I would say is not the most mentally tough person in the world. BUT, after three cycles of chemo on a nasty Lieomyosarcoma cancer, I was impressed by her will to live. It seems like we all have this ability to push through pain, sickness, fatigue, if we still have that will to keep going. I am a strong supporter of fitness during cancer treatments. It is tough to do, not fun all the time, but will challenge you to your core to keep fighting.

Our Navy SEAL creed has a few lines I say to help me push myself when fatigue sets in:

Never Quit — Never Fail — Never Out of the Fight

So keep fighting! One thing I do know though is that physical training programs will help your self-esteem and confidence, which is perhaps the first step to gaining mental toughness for some. But, Mental Toughness! How do you get it? Are you born with it? Can you acquire it?

Take for example, the five time Tour de France winner, Lance Armstrong who endured one of the toughest diseases by beating cancer. After his battle with cancer, he came back mentally tougher and has been at the top of his game ever since. Maybe he had it all along, who knows? Mental toughness is not measurable and is completely internal. But I believe hard work will get you there.

When Lance Armstrong was asked by reporters "What are you on?" referring to performance enhancing drugs. Lance stated, "I am on my BIKE — busting my ass for 6–8 hours a day!"

I have seen many great athletes not able to graduate SEAL training, and a few men who were not in great of shape able to finish through shear determination and daily gut checks. The few who graduate have a common trait of being able to "play with pain" and a mental determination never to quit on themselves or most importantly their classmates. Men who played team sports that require playing with pain, such as wrestling, football, and lacrosse, usually did quite well. Having a team to workout with is essential - that is why the Beat Cancer Boot Camp appeals to me and why the founder, Anita Kellman, uses Navy SEAL style workouts.

The key is to "live to compete, not to merely survive". This is the biggest difference in those who graduate any special forces training and those who do not. Whether you physically ace the pre-SEAL fitness test, or barely pass it, ALL depends on your mental toughness. In fact, finding humor in what happens to you daily is one of the best ways to get through the daily grind. Once again, being able to laugh about your cancer with friends is huge for your healing process.

In your journey to find mental toughness remember to train smart and not push yourself to injury that will require medical attention. Good luck and keep pushing through.

Chapter Four: For Health — Be A Control Freak

Being Proactive

Taking charge of your health is the most important first step. Even though there are certain circumstances beyond anyone's control, there are some things that can be done. Rule number one … don't be afraid to question. To question is to learn. You must realize you are an intelligent person who wants to make educated decisions.

Taking control of one's disease begins with just that, asking questions. You cannot take control with out knowing your options. Just as you would do research when you have to make a big purchase, or a life altering decision. You must learn and fully understand your alternatives. It's no different than when you are newly diagnosed. The first thing to do is, stop everything, think, and slowly learn about your disease and your options.

Many people believe being a control freak is a poor characteristic. I disagree! You must not see yourself as a victim and allow others to dictate what to do. One of the first mantras I preach is to get a copy of all your test results. Some doctors will frown upon it, and perhaps tell you they can't do it. Guess what? They are YOUR results and they belong to you.

Doctors sometimes don't like to share this with patients because it brings up more questions. With all the physician practices so busy these days, they don't find the adequate time it takes to explain things. If you are not comfortable with your doctor, it is okay to seek a second opinion. Remember, it is YOUR health at stake, and you must find someone with whom you are comfortable. You need to find the best doctor to work with you, one that you trust. You need a good physician, not a nice guy, or a friend.

A major part of taking control is to be proactive. Don't just sit back and wait for things to happen. It is not rocket science what to do to stay healthy. Actually it's pretty basic.

Don't smoke.
Don't drink. (OK in moderation)
Watch your diet.
Exercise.

These are all things we know, but don't seem to control. This is where the discipline comes in to play. Doing these four basic rules will help you take charge of your health. So many common diseases could be prevented or controlled if we just follow these four simple take-charge commandments.

When diagnosed with cancer it seems like the rug was suddenly pulled out from underneath. Life throws it's curve ball and you never saw it coming. This is the time you must begin to get all your recent test results. The results should be exact copies of the same ones your doctor received, not some generic letter. Once you have the test results in hand, you are empowered to ask the right questions to perform your research.

This day and age, all patients should be part of the decision making process of their treatment. That is the only way you can ensure that you will be comfortable with the plans, and ultimately satisfied with the results. No one should dictate to you what should be done. This is YOUR body and YOUR life. We all make choices. I understand that sometimes it may be uncomfortable to question your physician. Most likely, you were sent to a specialist because your primary doctor referred you. There would be no reason for anyone to have all kinds of surgeons, and oncologists on call for them! Remember, just because you were referred doesn't mean it is a mandatory assignment!

You will know if your specialists are a good fit once you begin asking questions. Some are very eager to answer and assist you, while others will be annoyed that you are questioning them. Each diagnosis is unique, and your treatment should be personalized. There are no two patients who can possibly have the exact disease. There are too many variables. The issue gets complicated if you start comparing yourself to others.

I have heard over and over. "Well my cousin had this cancer and her doctor did this…" or "My friend told me about this new treatment." It is perfectly fine to listen to others, as long as you keep in mind that no two diseases are identical. Knowledge is power and don't be afraid to pick the brain of everyone around you. Just remember to keep it in perspective.

Be as specific as you can when you ask questions. Asking general questions does not help you. This disease is all about you and each question should remain focused on you.

Share your experience with others. Don't be shy about telling people what happened to you, good or bad. Be honest and upfront. Keep in mind, you are not attempting to give medical advice. You are simply sharing your experience and the opinions they generated. Others will most likely thank you for sharing.

Recommended Elements of Physical Activity for Improving Cancer:

Achieve or maintain ideal body weight
Muscle strength and endurance
Flexibility exercises
Cardiovascular endurance
Restoration of functions for activities of daily life

Health benefits of exercise

Physical activity has been linked to improved survival and quality of life in cancer survivors. An alarming number of cancer survivors who gained weight (especially common in breast cancer patients) in their first year of diagnosis, had increased risk of recurrence and lowered risk of survival, compared to those who maintained pre-diagnosis weight. Physical activity can assist in weight control, among other benefits to the body and mind. Exercise not only improves the physical well-being, but also the mental, and social well-being. Physical activity offers a low-cost, non-pharmacological treatment option to lower the risk of cancer recurrence and death.

Because of these factors, physicians are increasingly recommending that cancer survivors participate in exercise routines as part of their recovery from cancer, and prevention of cancer recurrence. To gain all the benefits from being physically active, an exercise program should include flexibility, strength, and cardiovascular endurance.

Being physically flexible does not necessarily mean training to do the splits! The goal for flexibility is to have the joints in the body be able to move through a full range of motion. For example, rotate the shoulder in a full large circle. Being flexible allows the muscles in the body to bend and stretch frequently; decreasing the chance of injury, which often accompanies aging.

Muscular strength is important in an exercise program because it will assist in gaining lean muscle mass. Exercises that build muscle strength are simply ones that use resistance. Training with weights (heavier weights with less repetitions), or pushing against your own body weight alone can accomplish this goal. Strong core muscles (back and abdomen in particular) are important for posture and prevention of back injury.

Cardiovascular endurance incorporates using the body's large muscles at a moderate intensity, for an extended amount of time. Simply, 25–30 minutes of brisk walking 3–5 times/week can fulfill this requirement. Aerobic exercise is a form of cardiovascular endurance, and benefits include improved circulation, increased breathing efficiency, strengthening of the heart muscle, and reduced blood pressure.

Because breast cancer survivors have an increased risk of cardiovascular disease and diabetes, both conditions which recommend physical activity as part of the treatment, it is important that cancer survivors incorporate cardiovascular endurance as part of their program for preventing cancer recurrence. Like the benefits of cardiovascular endurance to cancer survivors, muscular endurance (lighter weight with more repetitions) can increase and/or maintaining bone density, which is particularly important for osteoporosis prevention.

Simply being able to stand up straight and walk with ease can improve the confidence of a cancer survivor. Feeling and looking physically strong improves self-image, which in return encourages social interactions, both of which improve quality of life. Boot camp training not only incorporates flexibility, muscular strength, and cardiovascular endurance, it offers companionship by bringing people together in a support group, and promoting social interactions. Boot camp training provides physical activity needed for cancer survivors, giving them the energy throughout the day, and strength to meet daily physical challenges and the demands in fighting cancer.

Boxes of Inspiration

Throughout the book you will see boxes of inspirational writings of many of the women who participate in the Beat Cancer Boot Camp. They are heart-felt recollections of their experiences with cancer and how exercise helped them cope with the daily grind of treatments, the illness, and a variety of other pressures that can overwhelm you. But, know that you are not alone and gain strength from those who have been there before you.

From Cancer Patient

I had taken a Boot Camp pamphlet from my doctor's office when I was newly diagnosed … just something to distract me while I waited to be called into the exam room. It looked interesting, but I was overwhelmed with everything being thrown at me, and definitely not the support group type. Plus, at 45, everyone in the waiting room was much older than I and would have no idea what a cancer diagnosis meant to a working woman with young children. It ended up at home in my junk mail pile for several months.

A couple of months into treatment, I felt like I was holding up pretty well. My husband, however, noticed that I was always sleeping on the couch and had become pretty isolated. He had been amazingly supportive but really felt I needed to talk to people who actually understood what I was going through. He suggested I join some sort of support group. I am not the support group type. A bunch of sad, cancer-stricken women sitting around with Kleenex boxes, sharing how scared they are and how badly treatment makes them feel, would surely only make me feel worse!

He reminded me about the Boot Camp pamphlet we had seen in the office months before, and I reluctantly agreed to check it out. I went to the website and RSVP'd to go to the lunch group … just this once.

As I walked apprehensively towards the private room at the back of the restaurant, I was preparing myself for a group of elderly, pale, bald, cancer patients and the awkward silence that comes with being the new person in a room where people are already emotionally connected. When I opened the door, I was sure the hostess had misunderstood me. The room was brimming with laughing, noisy, professionally dressed women, young and old, who didn't even look close to being dead! While we ate, they each introduced themselves, giving a brief history of their cancer diagnosis and their treatment regimens. These women were not victims. They had come to terms with the hand they had been dealt, and were attacking their challenges head-on with an incredible amount of contagious, positive energy.

As I listened to each survivor's story, I began to realize that cancer can only control your life if you give it that power. Of course you have to mourn your diagnosis, but you can't get stuck there. Whether I live a month or 50 more years, why waste a single day of it being angry and asking the proverbial "why me?

- Liz A.

Chapter Five: For Life — The Ripple Effect

Camaraderie

One evening I was out to dinner with my mother and two daughters. Sitting there, I was thinking how fortunate I was to be with three generations. It was a pleasant evening, and my daughters started talking about being sisters. My mother then started talking about her sister. The conversation went on and on about what a unique relationship sisters have. I enjoyed listening to all their stories, never giving it a second thought. Just smiling to myself how nice it was that we were all together.

All of a sudden, my mother said to us, that she was so sorry that she never had any more children. Perhaps if she did, she would have had another girl and I would have had a sister. Wow, that was pretty powerful to admit that to not only me, but my daughters. Truthfully, I never gave that a second thought, growing up the middle child with two brothers. To hear that my mother felt sad for me was kind of surprising.

As I was preparing for our anniversary event for Boot Camp I sat down to write my opening speech. I was so excited for the celebration – I could hardly wait. The evening was perfect. All the chairs were lined up, and filled. There was standing room only. As I approached the podium to deliver the welcome speech, I looked at the crowd and held back some tears. It was starting to sink in, what this group has become - not only to me, but the community.

I began my speech by welcoming all the guests and dignitaries who attended. I thanked my family for their continued support. I then looked at my mother, who was beaming from her seat, and continued my speech. I shared the story about the restaurant conversation from the night before. I'm sure no one knew where I was going with all this. I then looked at my mother and said, "Mom, you were so sad you never had any more children, so I could share those wonderful ties with a sister."

I then looked at all the Boot Camp gals in the audience, and said. "Will all my sisters please stand" There were so many people standing. I looked at my mother and said. "See Mom, don't be sad anymore, I do know what it's like to have sisters."

Over the years I realized that this is more than a program. This is a powerful sisterhood, bringing together people whose paths would have never crossed, if it wasn't for cancer. The closeness we have for each other is hard to describe. I started recognizing what I was doing with my life. Weeding out people who zapped my energy, and focusing it on people I truly cared about, Boot Camp members! It dawned on me that these are the important friends of my life that make a difference.

We are together 2–3 times a week, and share just about everything. The comfort level we have as a group is amazing. It is all about relationship building, which doesn't happen overnight. These are the people that any of us can call day or night, and we will be there for each other… no questions asked. How lucky that we have that. It is a secure feeling to know you are never alone. This group means so much too so many. Even with all our different personalities, quirks, religious and political opinions, there is a bond that can't be broken.

We have shared losses together. An original Boot Camp member passed away recently. Not many people in today's group actually knew her. The group has grown so much since its inception, and Kathy wasn't around much due to her illness. A very active member and her best friend, Ginny, continued to come to classes. When Ginny needed us in time of support to help her through this very difficult process, we were all there for her. Not because they knew Kathy, but because they know Ginny. Never leave a troop member in need.

The camaraderie we find with each other is more than skin deep. By that I mean it is worn on the outside, whether it's newest camo attire or other Boot Camp accessories. It is important for everyone to feel part of the group. This new strong, tough persona is one everyone embraces.

This is why members always seem to enjoy sharing their new discoveries with each other. Watching their faces beam with excitement like they just found the best treasure.

One day I was talking about how we were going to have promotional DVD made, to promote the program. I explained that they would be filming our group in action, because we all know action speaks louder than words, and they would all get to be part of the story. The excitement was building.

A few days later, in walks a Boot Camp member with a surprise for me. It was a camo director's chair, with my name "Sarge" embroidered on it, just like you see in the movies. I was deeply touched by this. Not only did she make it for me to enjoy, but this contribution showed the connection she felt to the program. It was her way of saying thanks.

I remembered the first day Kathy walked into a Boot Camp class. I previously met her at the office I was working at. She had just gone undergone a bilateral mastectomy, and was feeling all alone. Nearing retirement, this was just another change in her life she didn't know if she could handle. I encouraged her to come by the class, just to meet the women, hoping her spirits would be boosted.

To my disappointment, when she showed up, she walked over to the group, and quickly turned away in tears. To be truthful, I never had this reaction before from anyone and didn't quite know how to take it. I contacted her soon after, and talked about what happened. When she felt ready to return she did. She did what she could in class and didn't feel alone anymore. Always wearing Boot Camp attire and a smile on her face, she knew now she had a home with Boot Camp. The gift of the director's chair, showed me her appreciation, pointing her in the right direction.

At one of our holiday gatherings, we were busy setting up the tables for our brunch. Arranging the camo tablecloths and place settings is part of our ritual. Pam C., who is the fashion maven of the group was working at a boutique at this time. In she walks with dozens of cute little gift bags, filled with a surprises. I help her place one at each place setting, for this was her gift to the women. As we all sit around the tables together, and begin with the introductions, everyone was anxious to see what was in those little gift bags. On the count of three, we were all able to open them up at the same time, and out comes camo thongs!! Some of the gals quickly put them on … their heads! The laughter and look on their faces was hilarious. Nothing surprises us from Pam, the bling queen.

Carol M. started attending Boot Camp class years ago. A single mom with a teenager, she's a very dedicated member. I believe Carol was looking for other women she could feel empowered by. She might be quiet in class but is always volunteering ways to help. She loves to sew, and is creative. One day I requested to have some beanbags for some exercises, and in no time I had dozens ready to go. You guessed it, camo bean bags! We were planning some trips, and she designed... camo luggage tags. Oh, and those camo table cloths that we use, she was not happy with the way I just took a scissors and cut the nylon parachutes to fit the tables. She took them home and seamed them. It's the pride that she has in feeling part of a group she belongs to that is important.

Margo, a buddy, joined the group and felt she wanted to give back in some way. Little did I know how much she enjoyed being part of Boot Camp, that she even talked to her family about it.. Her dad, an avid garage-sale hunter, went on a mission to find camo attire and boots at various yard sales. Shortly after, Margo proudly comes walking up to the group with two big boxes filled with pants, jackets, and boots. Now everyone has the opportunity to dress the part. When I thanked her for her donation, she said it was the least she could do, and that her father enjoyed his mission … to help Boot Camp!

Everyone is always on the look-out for any camo accessory. From various clothing items, hats, scarves, cool neck ties to wear in the hot summer months — even custom drapes over the windows. There is always something new added to our collection. I believe this more than an attitude. This is part of belonging to a group, and feeling part of something. It gives everyone a chance to find strength and courage and to become someone they have never been. Someone a little bit stronger than they were before. Dressing the part, in their tough Boot Camp attire even if it's only for one hour, their image changes and so does their attitude. They earned bragging rights … they are now part of Boot Camp. It shows inside and out.

Connections, Bonds

Not withstanding the continual excitement of Boot Camp growth, change is always difficult. We recently experienced this with a pivotal member of the group, who jumped in feet first and had an impact on almost everyone she met.

Ro joined Boot Camp after relocating here from New York. She felt lost in our community but quickly found her niche with us. She was able to always bring joy and laughter to the group. We never knew exactly what would come out of her mouth. Some things would shock us at first, but after all, we are a diverse group of women, and we could handle almost anything we heard.

The one thing that we all found difficult was when she announced she was relocating back to New York. We could handle almost anything … but trying to imagine Boot Camp without Ro? This can't be happening. We all tried to convince her in various ways to break the deal, and stay with us, her other family. What touched me most by this is everyone felt the same way. The closeness we have with one another is unique.

What I began to observe is that she started distancing herself from the group the moment she announced her move. Gone were the days in which she would show up for every class, dinner, lunch or activity. After giving this some thought, I called her. It took some time for her to return my calls. I knew what was happening. I finally came out and asked if she was pulling away from the group because it was hard for her to leave us. She answered of course that was true. She said she couldn't bear the thought of not being part of the group, so it would be best to get use to it now. I told her, she is thinking of this all backwards. She is losing everyday she has with us. Not living in the moment, worrying about the future and trying to protect her feelings. Don't give up today for what tomorrow might bring.

The Buddy System

It's natural to feel uncertainly and fear joining a group all alone. It is sometimes very challenging to take that first step. This is where the buddy system comes in. It is a very simple but important concept. Buddies can be family or friends. Buddies can be people from the community who want to be there for others. Buddies are an important link to our success. Some people join up as a buddy, and can be assigned with a survivor. Some might come with a friend. A buddy provides motivation, encouragement and support.

A good buddy is hard to find … except at Boot Camp.

We had a newly diagnosed boot camp member whose friend dragged her to class. She really wasn't all that interested in the whole exercise thing. She was still kind of numb with her diagnosis. Like many others before her, she just didn't get it yet. Didn't understand how it could happen to her, when she felt so good. She really didn't know what was in store for her. Neither did her friend. She was just trying her best to be the best buddy there is, supporting her in every way. That is the only thing you can really do, because you just feel helpless.

They were both smart enough to know that with chemotherapy comes hair loss. That is almost as hard as losing the breast. To try to make her feel she's not alone, her friend arranged for a very special night out. They met at a beauty salon, which was closed to the public. A few family and friends gathered, and had some wine.

Then the big moment came for this survivor to take charge of her life. If you're going to lose your hair damn it, let's beat it to the punch line. So out came the clippers, and they shaved her head. To show solidarity, her friend joined right in and buzzed her hair as well! I wasn't there to witness this, but I know it must have been very emotional.

We watched them come to class together, week after week, smiling and being so proud of their connection with each other. Feeling strong and now confident they will be able to overcome this together. Best buddies.

Family Member with Cancer

In October of 2006, my family received the devastating news that my mom was diagnosed with breast cancer. She would not only have to endure a mastectomy, but chemotherapy and radiation. Mom, one of the bravest women I know, remained high-spirited throughout all of the struggles that were to come. Despite her admirable optimism and positive attitude, I knew that she had to be experiencing one of the toughest emotional battles of her life.

Even though my family was always there for her with the love and compassion, there was a certain amount of empathy and understanding that we could not share. That was when my sister found Boot Camp and suggested that mom try it. Soon afterwards, mom asked me to go with her for her first day of Boot Camp. Of course, I was thrilled to share in this experience and also excited to get a day of "easy exercise" underway. Little did I know …

Mom and I went to her first day of BCBC, and the women welcomed her with open arms and so much warmth. Then the warmth was kissed goodbye when Anita called the troops to the field! The squats, push-ups, jumping jacks, sprints and many more exercises began. I was in utter SHOCK! Here I am, a 24-year old girl who could not for the life of me keep up with these amazing women who have battled cancer. As the workout came to an end, and I could no longer feel my legs, I realized that this group of women was perfect for my mom.

These women do not feel sorry for themselves, and they do not feel powerless. They are powerful, optimistic, and astonishing women who support each other in every way imaginable. They share everything from the latest medical information to their emotional roller coasters that they endure throughout their battles.

These are the women who have supported mom in ways that my family could not. When mom comes home each time from BCBC with a smile on her face and muscles on her arms, I feel a sense of relief knowing that she has found the support that she needed and slightly jealous that she has found a way to look better than me!

- Shannon J.

Buddy of Cancer Patient

In July 2005, a childhood friend died of ovarian cancer. She lived in Austin, Texas, and moved back to our hometown of Los Angeles after diagnosis. She died 18 months after a valiant battle. Tania had an incredible presence and life force and was determined to survive but was unable to turn her fate around. I felt so helpless — helpless that I couldn't change her path and that I lived so far away. When another friend was diagnosed with breast cancer in December 2006, I was determined to do something, anything to make a difference.

I've known Anita since my family and I moved from LA to Tucson in 1992. She generously embraced us and became a part of our lives. I knew about Breast Cancer Boot Camp from its start. I always thought I'd go, but always had a million excuses not to. After my friend Tania's death, I started going to Boot Camp. I told myself it was to get in shape but truthfully I needed to heal from Tania's death and emotionally make up for not being there for her. I had my own selfish reasons — I wanted to feel better about myself.

When my friend Karen was diagnosed with cancer, I decided it was time to look outside myself and do something that could make a difference. At first I felt determined to be the best buddy ever. I went twice a week, suffered the tough — and I mean tough — workout and walked away feeling I was not only doing something for myself but for others. Then in time, I felt embarrassed. Embarrassed that I didn't have cancer and was trying to support people who had suffered beyond my personal experience. By being there, was I mocking them by my good health, my good fortune? I don't know why I gave into these insecurities, but I stopped going. Then I started making excuses, saying I was lazy. What a fool I was!

I woke up one day and realized that I can make a difference, and no one felt put off because I wasn't "one of them." Talk about twisting reality.

I love Boot Camp and what it represents. It represents life and living to the fullest. It brings women of all ages, sizes and experience together to share the good, bad and the ugly with humor and love. It has taught me that cancer for some is not the end, it's the beginning of seeing the world more clearly — embracing the good not dwelling in self-pity. This group of dynamic women are moving forward and not looking back. Bless Anita for making this happen and challenging all of us to never give up.

- Nancy V.

Pay it Forward – Giving back to the community

Being an active group in the community is the best outreach program you can have, and it feels good to be able to give back to others. Members won't see themselves as victims of a disease, but rather as ambassadors to healthy living. It is a great way to share your enthusiasm with others. If you have a group, make your presence known in the community!

Funny how quickly things change from searching for ways to get involved in the community to fielding calls from all over, wanting your group to participate. Hmmm, could it be that we are vibrant, fun, confident, and enthusiastic? Not your typical cancer support group that people are used to seeing. Wherever we go, and any functions we attend, we always wear our uniforms. They may not remember out names, but they remember the fatigues and combat boots. What an image — one that portrays strength and wellness. Studies have shown that attitude plays a role in recovery. What could be a better attitude than that? After we learn that giving feels better than receiving, we all tend to want to give back in some way.

Impact on Families and Friends

It is sometimes hard for people to really know how they can support and help their friends who are fighting cancer. They always mean well, but don't have the adequate words or experience to make a difference. That's another good reason to get involved in the community, because many troopers join Boot Camp on their family's encouragement. I've met many people at various races, events, or speaking engagements who have gone home and told family members or friends about this program. People often realize they know someone who would benefit from Beat Cancer Boot Camp, someone who's not destined for the typical support group.

Being part of this program opens it all up. What a relief for friends to see a loved one's strength and self-esteem rise so quickly. Family members have told me that our program has not only changed their thinking about cancer, but made them realize the inner strength they have. A young son once told his mother that Boot Camp made her so strong that there was nothing she couldn't get through. He was relieved that his mother was getting stronger, physically and mentally.

Boot camp for many is a family affair. Like any other commitments, you really need your family support to be able to attend all the workouts, and events. It sometimes does interfere with family activities, but they do see what a difference it is making. So they gladly support it. For many of the charity walks and outreach projects we do, it is nice to see family and friends walking side by side. They understand the importance and show their support.

The major thing I see, is not only the support physically, but knowing the importance of the emotional support. When I hear from a husband that he notices a change in the attitude of his wife, and she needs to come back for a Boot Camp "fix," I feel great. You know what they say: "A happy mom makes a happy home."

Protecting

As mothers, it is second nature to protect our families. That's what we do best. Remain strong. All of a sudden it hits you — why are you disappointed when family members aren't reaching out to you like you think they should? Could it be that you have created this wall around yourself to isolate and protect others who you don't think are strong enough to handle the situation? The problem arises when you are then hurt and disappointed not to be given the care and empathy you desire.

The most obvious solution, although might not be easy, is to be willing to share your feelings with others. This was a real eye opener for Loretta, who recently attended a Boot Camp retreat. She loves spending time with her family, so she invited her daughter to join her on our annual retreat. What quality mother-daughter time to be spent together! How wonderful that her daughter will see how strong and inspiring her mother is to others.

I know Loretta was excited not only to share this retreat with her daughter, but also to show her daughter the camaraderie of Boot Camp. Her daughter was able to get to know others as we sat around at various times just chatting. This was not a "let's sit around in a circle and share stories." This was more Boot Camp style, informal and talking about everything and anything whenever we had a moment.

On the second evening we were together at a dinner show, Loretta shared with the group something that happened to her during her treatment. Her astounded daughter turned around and with tears in her eyes, gave her mom a hug, and said, "Mom, I never realized what you went through." You see, Loretta was one of those strong moms, protecting her family by keeping everything from them. She thought she was doing the right thing, but at that "Aha" moment in her life, she suddenly realized it was her own actions that sheltered her family from the truth. Consequently, she never received the necessary support from them.

"Obstacles don't have to stop you. If you run into a wall, don't turn around and give up. Figure out how to climb it, go through it, or work around it."

- Michael Jordan

Chapter Six: Basic Training – Warm up and Stretch

Getting Started
The following stretching plan will assist you with getting started again safely and without as much post-exercise soreness.

The Stretching Program (FULL BODY STRETCH)
Increasing one's flexibility should be the first goal before starting a fitness program. In fact, if you are thinking about beginning a fitness program and you have been idle for many years, you should stretch for an entire week prior to starting running, lifting weights, or doing any calisthenics exercise. It is OK to walk to warm up however. So, your first 1–2 weeks of starting a fitness program should consist of the following stretches 1–2 times a day, drinking 2–3 liters of water a day, and walking, biking or some other non-impact low intensity cardio activity for 10–15 minutes.

Stretching and Warming Up/Cooling Down
A brief, full-body warm up will get the blood pumping and make sure the muscle are ready to be stretched. Biking, jogging, jumping jacks, a few pushups or crunches are all good for a warm up.

Stretch in this order to aid in major muscle group stretching. Stretching the connecting groups of the thighs and hamstrings first will assist in a more thorough stretch of the hams and thighs — the major muscle groups of the body. Hold these stretches or do these movements for at least 15–20 seconds each.

Follow the stretching chart after your main workout, too. Do not bounce when performing these stretches and inhale deeply for three seconds, hold for three seconds and fully exhale. This will take you to the 15–20 second time minimum for optimal results.

The Stretching Chart

Jumping Jacks
Press-Press Fling
Shoulder Shrugs
Arm/Shoulder Stretch
Chest/Bicep/Shoulder/Back Stretch
Shoulder Rotations
Tricep/Back Stretch (half moon)
Cobra Stretch
Mid back - Cat Stretch
Lower back Stretch #1,2
ITB/Hip
Down Dog Pose
Hamstring Stretch
Thigh Stretch — standing of laying on floor
Yoga Lunge
Calf Stretch

— See pictures and descriptions of each with our troops performing them in the following pages

When you are in doubt of what you can do for a workout. Try to do the stretches each day. You will feel better after a 10–15 minute stretch following the stretch guide on the following pages:

Explanation of the Stretches

Jumping Jacks — Warm up with jumping jacks or slow jog to get the blood flowing to your muscles. Take about 2–3 minutes doing 2–3 sets of 20–30 jumping jacks.

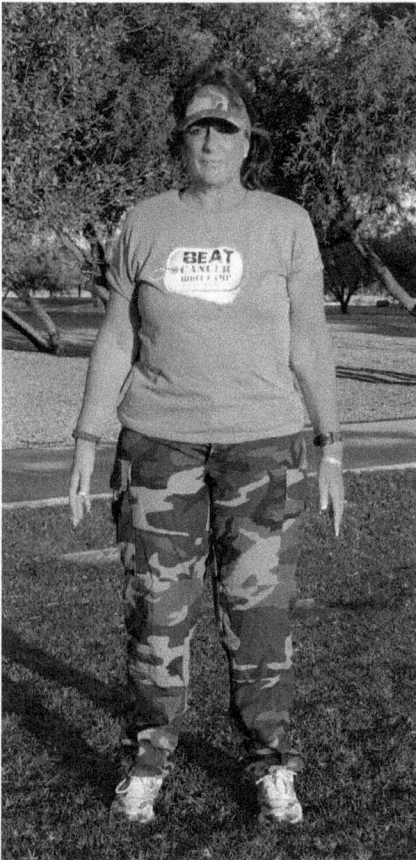

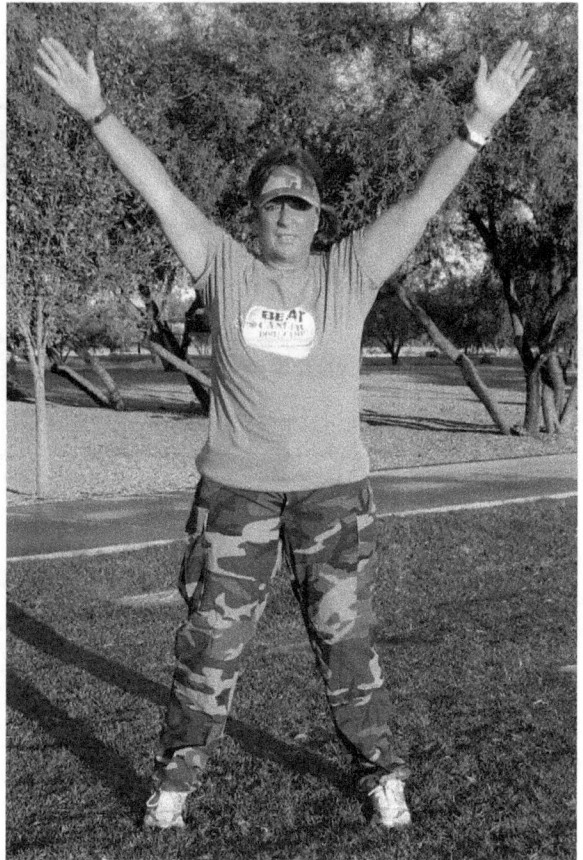

Name: Pam Chess Age: 58
Survivor: (type): Breast, # years: 5 ½ years
How long in BCBC: 5 ½ years
Occupation: Retired
Something of Interest: Tennis, Painting, my grandkids Shaelyn & Georgi
and Boot camp!!

Press - Press and Fling - Chest Stretch — Lift both arms in front of you and pull them back like you were doing a pushup two times. Then on the third, "fling" your arms back like you were doing a chest fly.

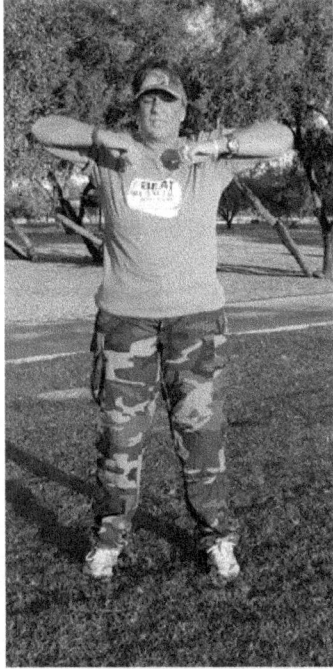

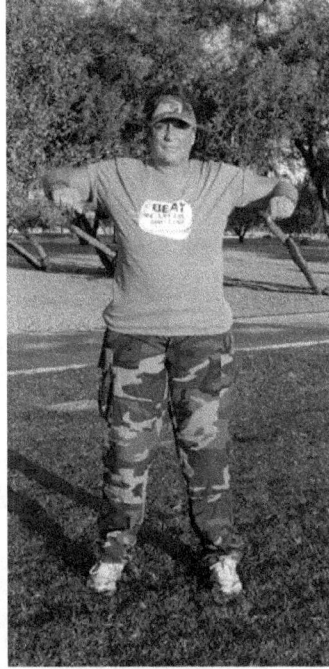

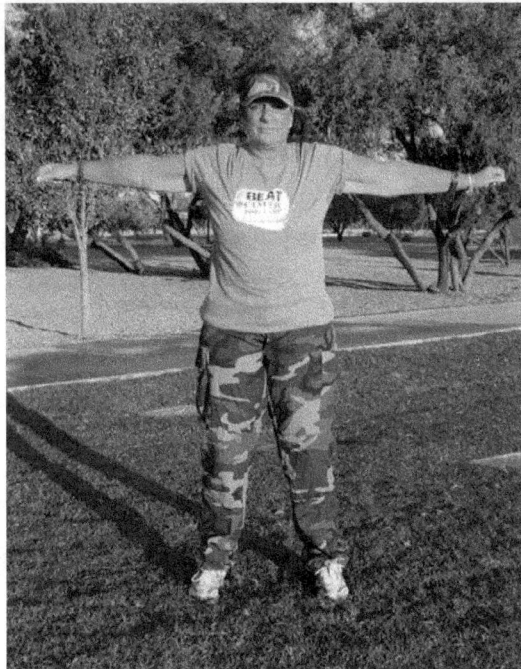

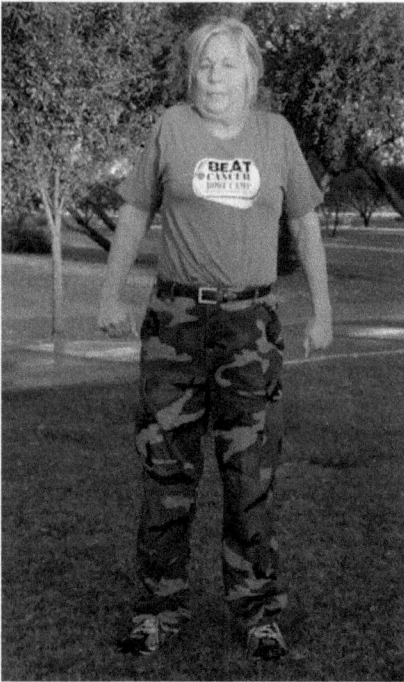

Arm / Shoulder Circles — Rotate your shoulders slowly in big circles forward and reverse for 15 seconds each direction.

Name: Marlyne Freedman
Age: 62
Buddy
How long in BCBC: 3 yrs
Something of Interest: I have 2 sons and 5 grandchildren. I have been a non-profit professional for over 30 years. I enjoy new challenges!

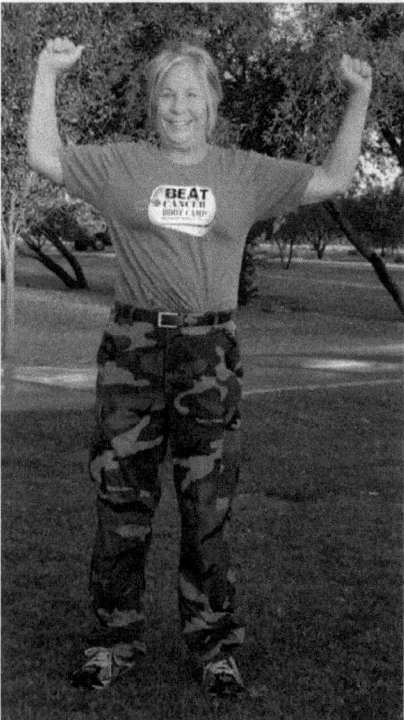

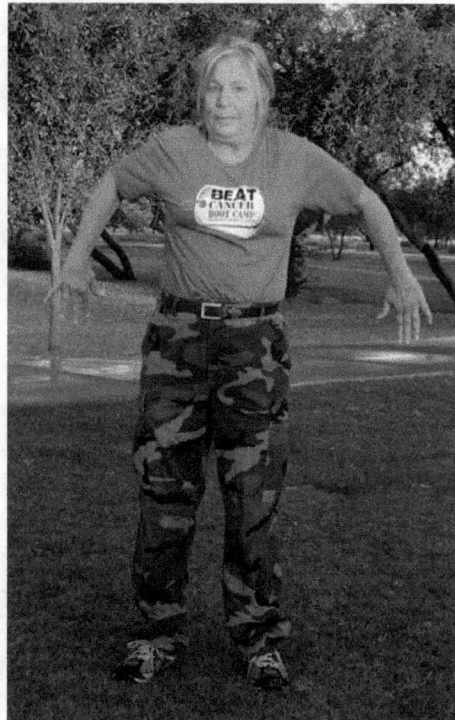

Shoulder Rotations — This movement helps warm up the rotator cuff and shoulder joint. It's a great one to do if you are about the throw a ball or just need to work on full range of motion of the shoulder

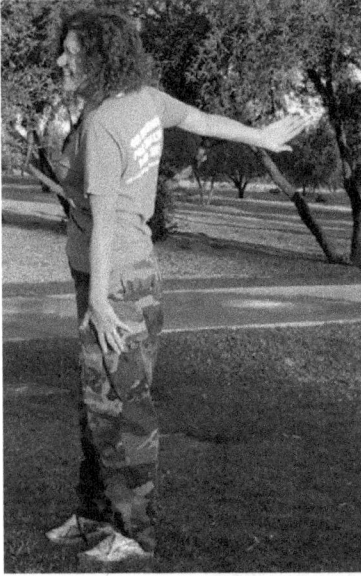

Chest / Shoulder / Upper Back Stretch — Grab onto a pole or wall and twist opposite of your arm until you feel the stretch in your chest and shoulder connection.

Option two, the swimmer stretch: Grab your hands behind your back and pull your shoulders back standing upright with chest out. Then roll the shoulders forward and take chin to chest.

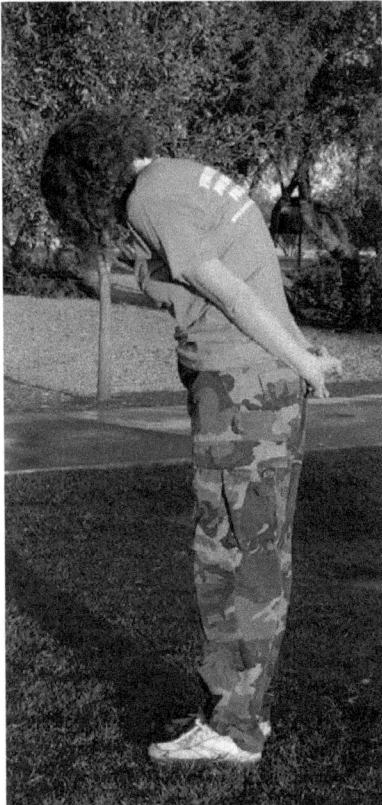

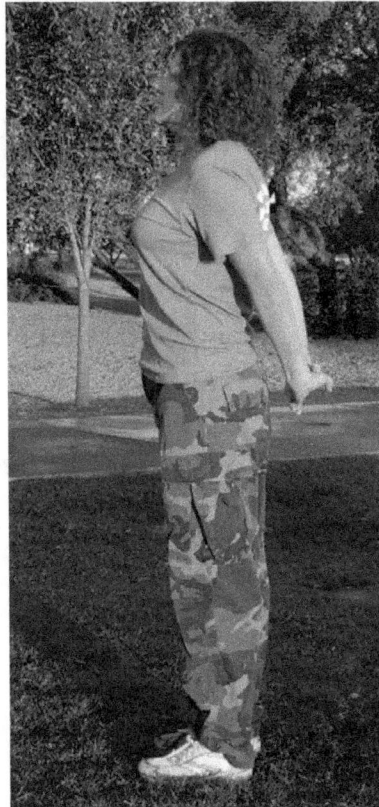

Arm Shoulder Stretch — Grab arm with opposite arm and pull it across the body stretching the rear shoulder and upper back. Rotate hands with thumbs down. Rotate.

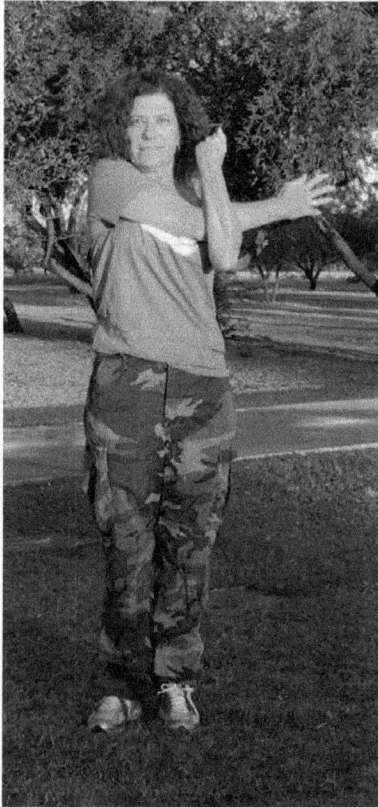

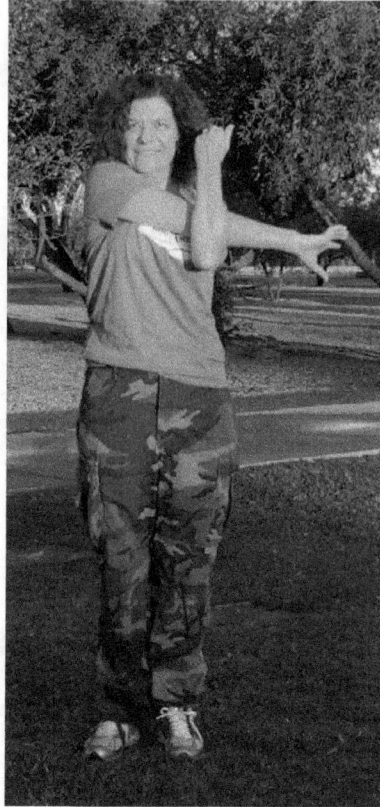

Name: Nancy Vornholt
Age: 54
Buddy
How long in BCBC: 3 years
Occupation: Project Manager
Something of Interest:
Wonderful husband and 2 children. Great at ping-pong!

Triceps into Back Stretch — Place both arms over and behind your head. Grab your right elbow with your left hand and pull your elbow toward your opposite shoulder. Lean to the side with each pull. Repeat with the other arm.

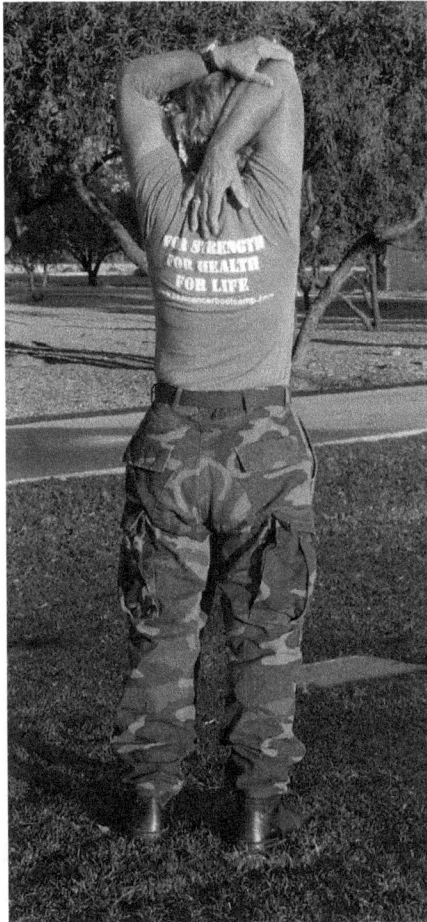

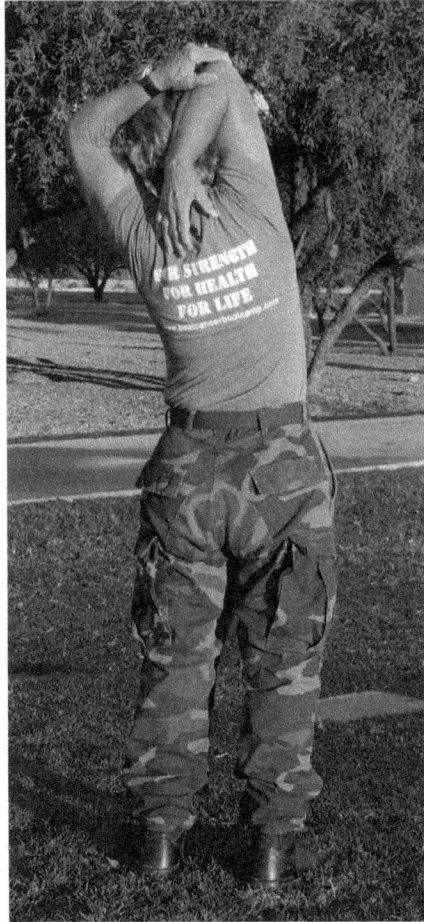

Name: Shirley Ruane
Age: 73
Survivor: (type): Breast # years: 13 years
How long in BCBC: 1 year
Occupation: Tennis Coach/Instructor
Something of Interest: Hiking, Kayaking, Birding

Abdominal Stretch — Lie on your stomach. Push yourself up to your elbows. Slowly lift your head and shoulders and look up at the sky or ceiling. Hold for 15 seconds and repeat two times.

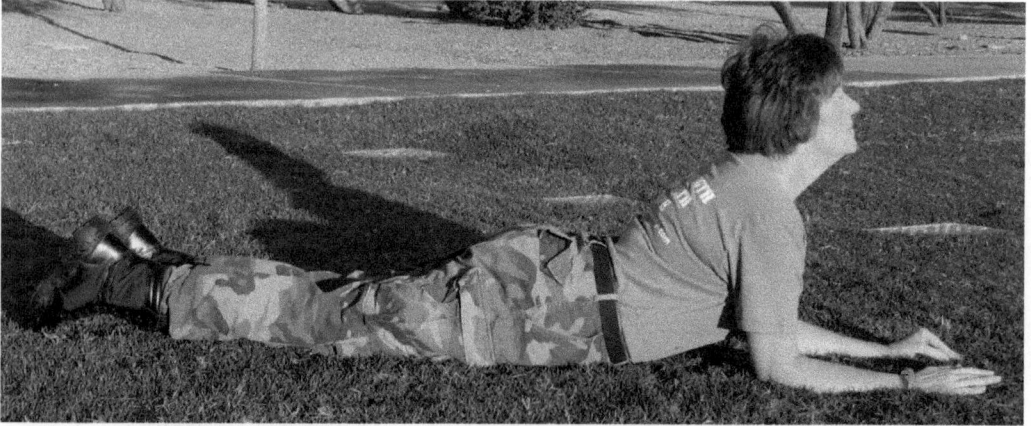

Back Stretch #1 – Cat Stretch — Get on all fours as shown and bow your back. Try to keep your head as close to your shoulders as possible. Put your chin to your chest and hold for 10 seconds.

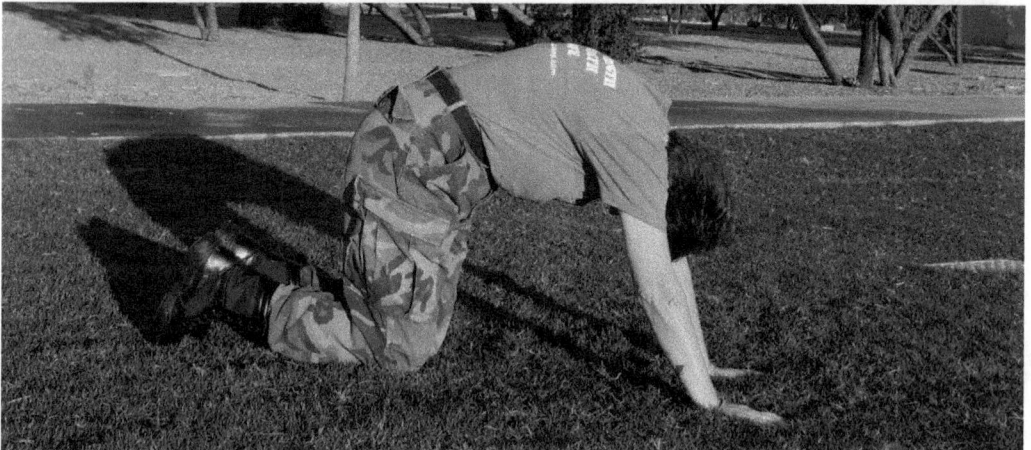

Name: Karen O'Brien
Age: 48
Survivor: (type): Breast # years: 3 years
How long in BCBC: 3 years
Occupation: Accountant
Something of Interest: I have a wonderful husband and three fabulous kids who are the center of my life! When I was in my 20s I jumped out of airplanes.

Back Stretch #2 — Lie on your left side. Place your top leg in front of you. Slowly twist your torso until your shoulders touch the floor. Hold for 15 seconds and repeat on the right side.

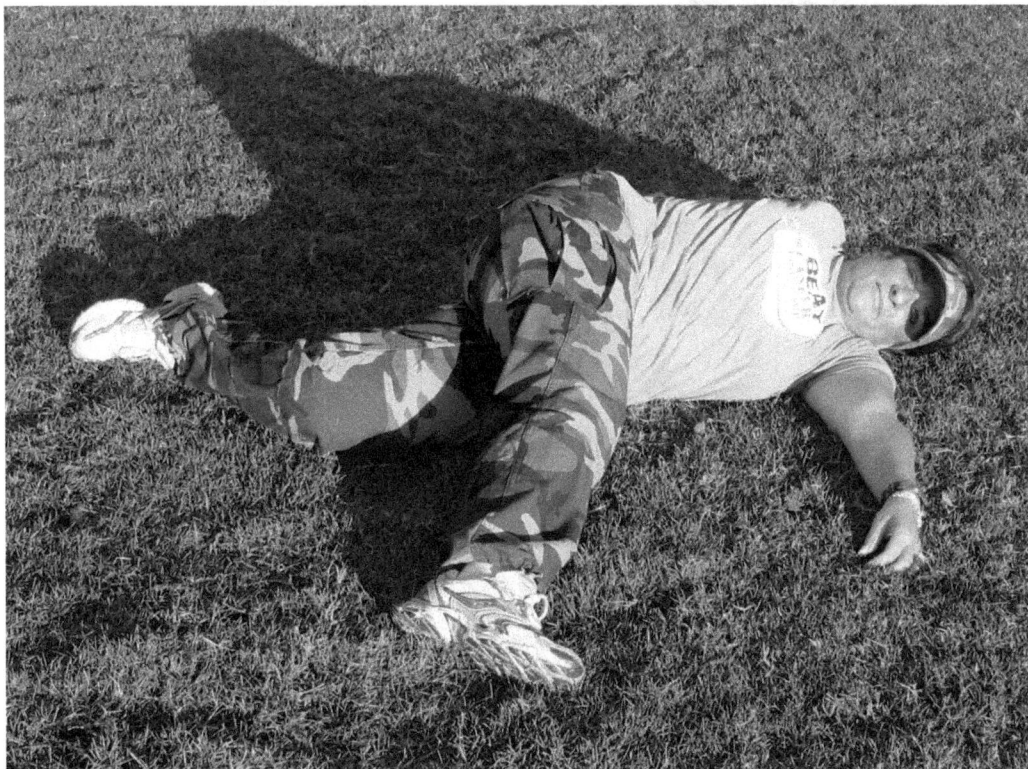

Name: Pam Chess
Age: 58
Survivor: Breast # years: 5 1/2
How long in BCBC: 5 1/2 years
Occupation: Retired
Something of interst: Tennis, painting, my grandkids, Shaelyn &
Georgi and Boot Camp

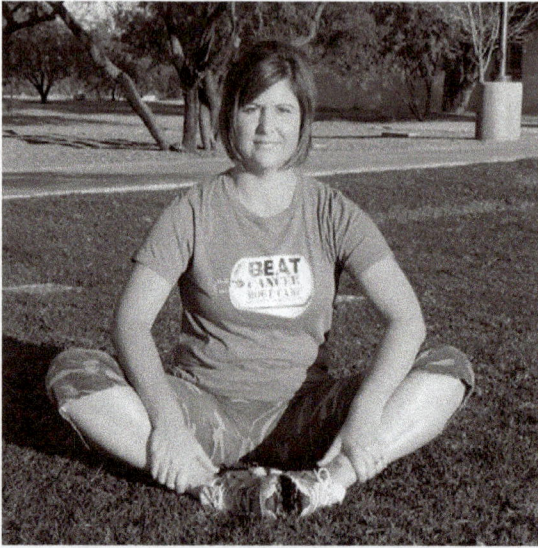

Butterfly stretch #1/#2 — Sitting with legs bent in front of you, stand so the heels of your feet touch and bring them as close to your body as you can. Try to stretch by opening your leg further — NO NEED TO PRESS on your legs to open.

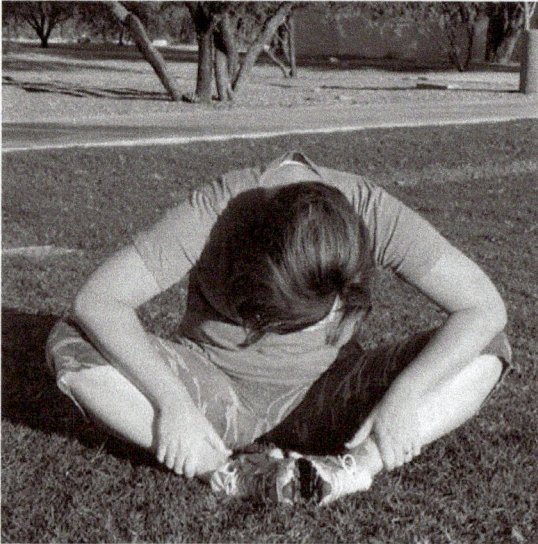

Butterfly stretch #1/#2 — Slightly straighten your legs about one foot but keep your feet touching and try to take your head in between your knees.

The lower back/hip connection is one of the most commonly injured areas of the body. Many lower back problems stem from inactivity, lack of flexibility, and improper lifting of heavy objects. Stretching and exercising your lower back will help prevent some of those injuries.

Name: Erin Resnick
Age: 36
Buddy
Occupation; Stay at home mom
Something of interest: I love spending time with my friends and family.
Boot Camp is fun and challenging, and I look forward to it.

Hip/outer thigh stretch (ITB) — Sit down with your left leg crossed over your right leg. Grab the left leg with both hands around the thigh / shin (with leg bent) and pull toward your chest, then twist. Repeat with the other leg.

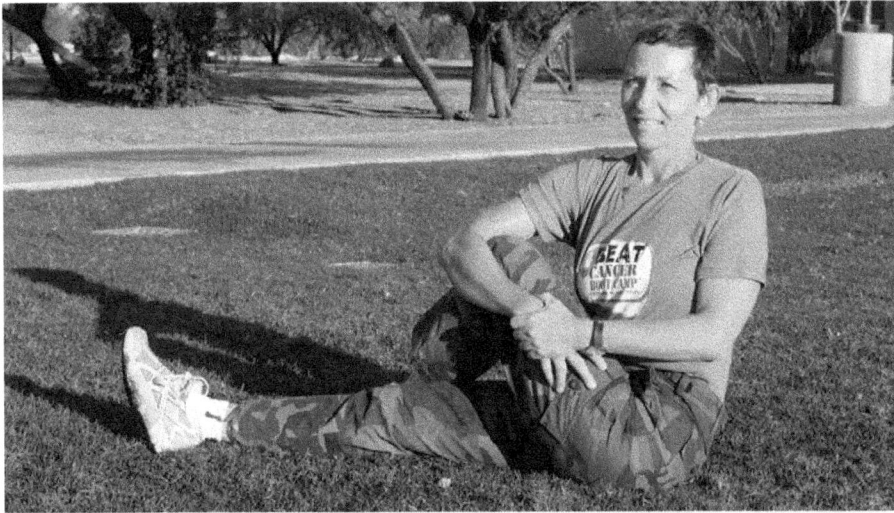

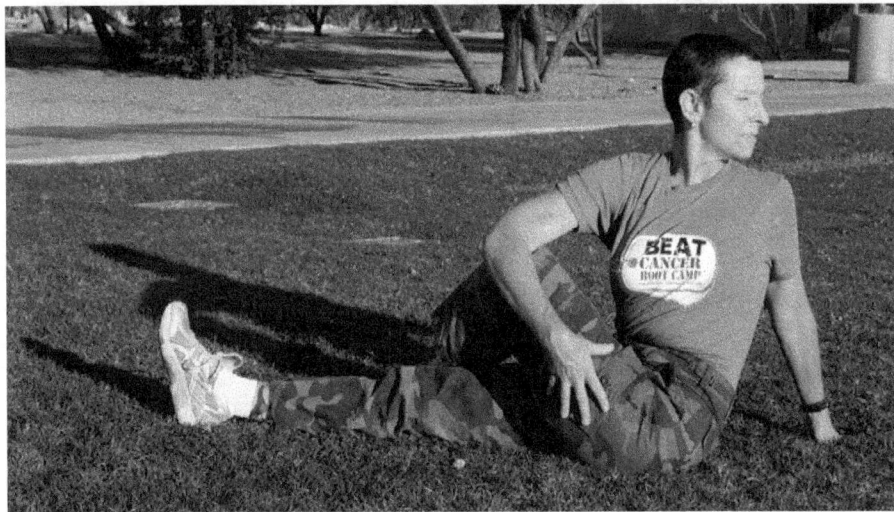

Name: Shawn Mulligan
Age: 47
Survivor: breast
How long in BCBC: 4 months
Occupation: Nurse
Something of interest: Cycled 250 miles with my family friends and our small kids along the Erie Canal in NY!

Down Dog Pose — Stretch the back of the legs and lower back with this relaxing yoga pose. Hold for 15-30 seconds. Try to keep your heels on the floor. NOTE — Try using this stretch to get up off the floor after doing a pushup — by slowly walking your hands toward your feet and standing.

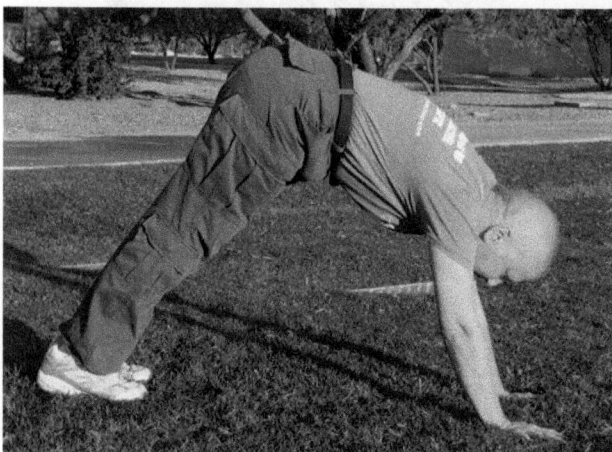

Yoga Lunge — Here is a tough hamstring exercise I recommend you do very slowly. Spread your legs as if you were doing a lunge and then take your torso to your front leg so you can place your hands to the floor as shown. Then slowly try to straighten the leg while keep your hands off the floor. Do this up-and-down motion 4-5 times and change legs for a thigh pump and hamstring stretch.

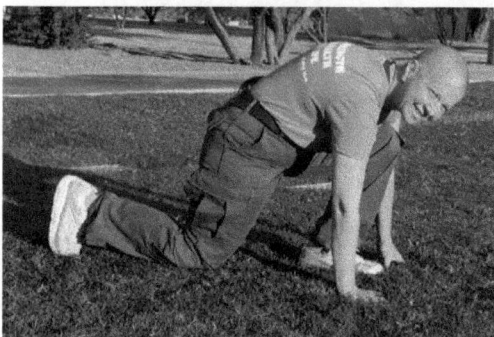
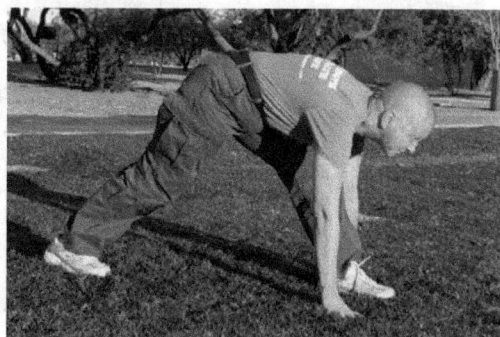

Name: Annie O'Connor
Age: 48
Survivor: (type): Breast
How long in BCBC: 3 months
Occupation: Speech Pathologist
Something of Interest: Interested in peace and social justice

Hamstring Stretch — From the standing or sitting position, bend forward at the waist and touch your toes. Keep your back straight and slightly bend your knees. You should feel this stretching the back of your thighs.

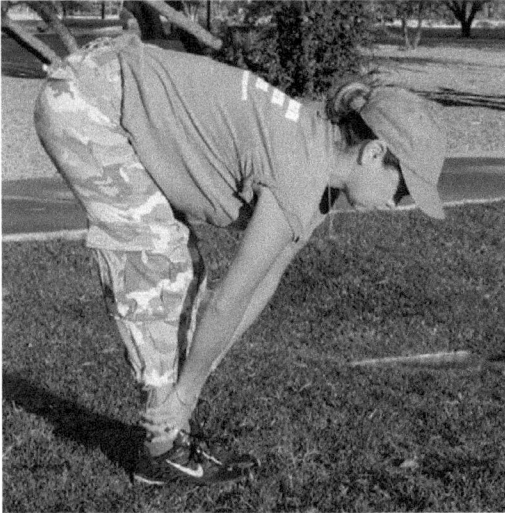

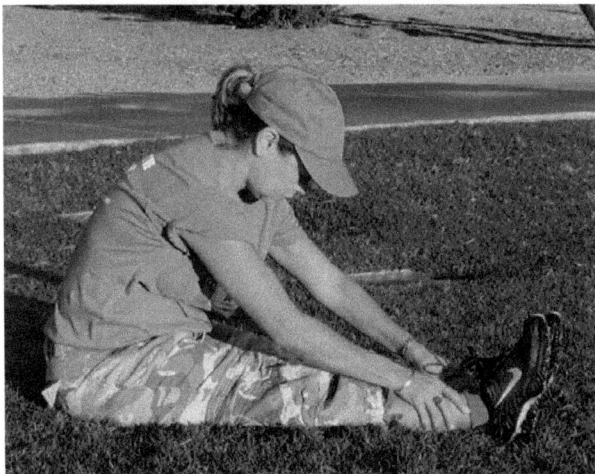

Name: Vianca Villa
Age:39
Buddy
Occupation: Case manager
How long in BCBC: 3 months
Something f interest: I enjoy doing yoga of which I have practiced
for over 4 years and I love the challenge of boot camp!

Thigh Stretch Standing — Standing, bend your knee and grab your foot at the ankle. Pull your heel to your butt and push your hips forward. Squeeze your butt cheeks together keep your knees close together. Hold for 10-15 seconds and repeat with the other leg. (You can hold onto something for balance if necessary, or you can lie down on your hip and perform this stretch.)

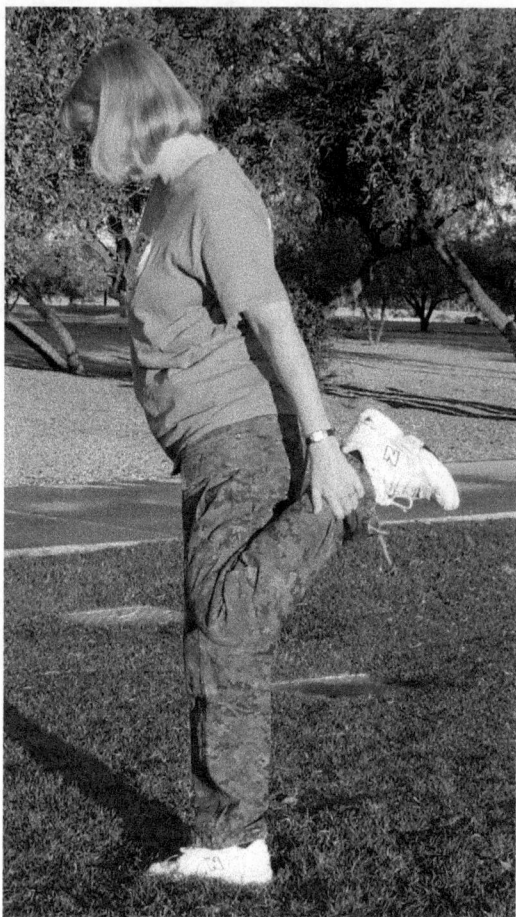

Name: Jenny Waters
Age: 51
Buddy
How long in BCBC: 5 years
Occupation: Archaeologist
Something of interest: Love the Blues and music in general

Calf Stretch into Achilles Tendon Stretch — Stand with one foot 2-3 feet in front of the other. With both feet pointing in the same direction as you are facing, put most of your body weight on your leg that is behind you — stretching the calf muscle. Now, bend the rear knee slightly. You should now feel the stretch in your heel. This stretch helps prevent Achilles tendonitis, a severe injury that will sideline most people for about 4–6 weeks.

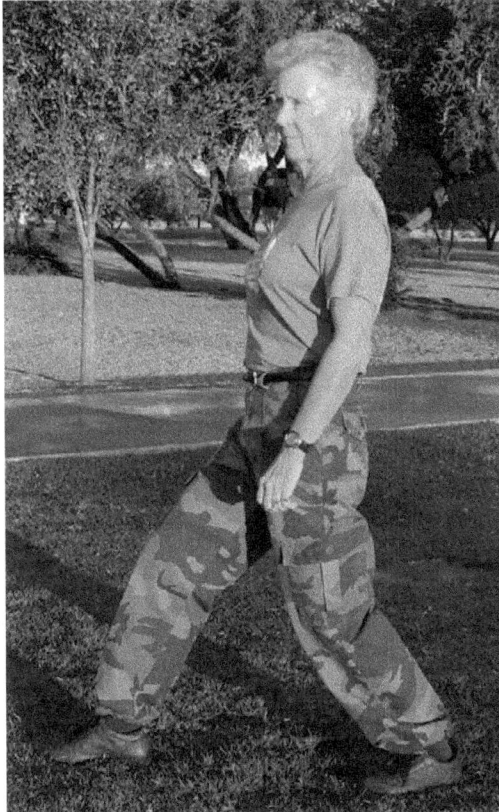

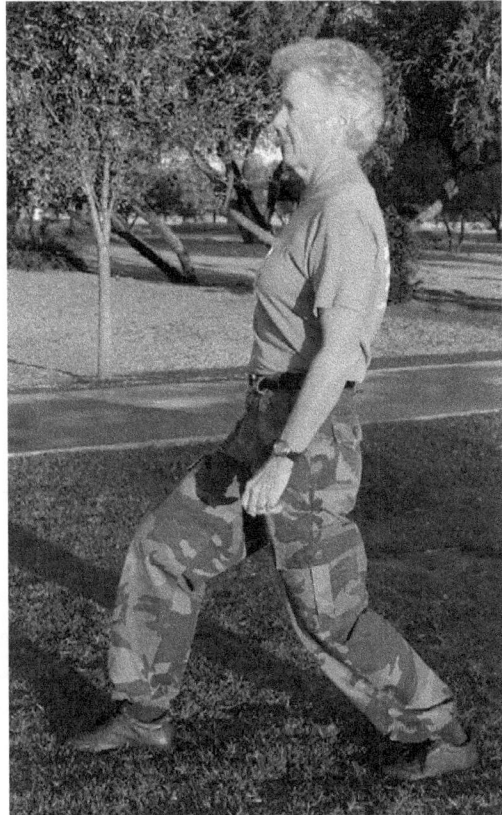

Name: Joanne Gouldin
Age: 56
Survivor: (type): Breast # years: New- I month
How long in BCBC: 1 month
Occupation: Insurance Account Executive
Something of Interest: Enjoy golf, walking

Chapter Seven: The Program
Lower Body Exercises

Squats — Keep your feet shoulder width apart. Drop your butt back as though sitting in a chair. Concentrate on squeezing your glutes in your upward motion. Keep your heels on the ground and knee over your ankles. Your shins should be vertical at all times. Extend your buttocks backward. While in the full-squat position, hold the pose and push yourself up and down within a 6 inch range of motion … just like riding a horse. Works the gluts, quads, and hams.

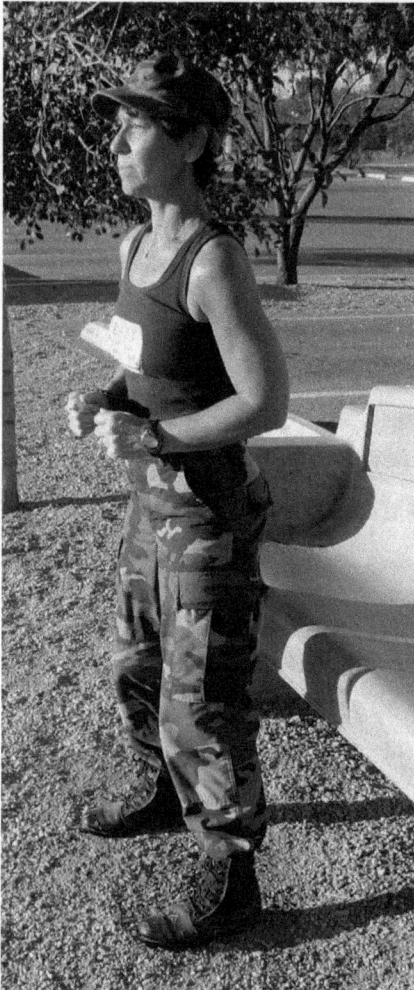

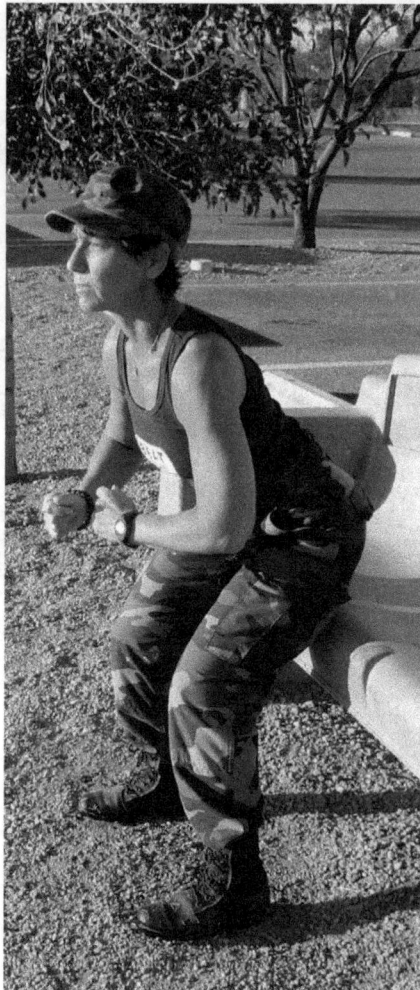

The One-Legged Squat — Intensify your squat by doing the squat on one leg. While in the full-squat position, hold the pose and push yourself up and down within a 6 inch range of motion. … just like riding a horse.

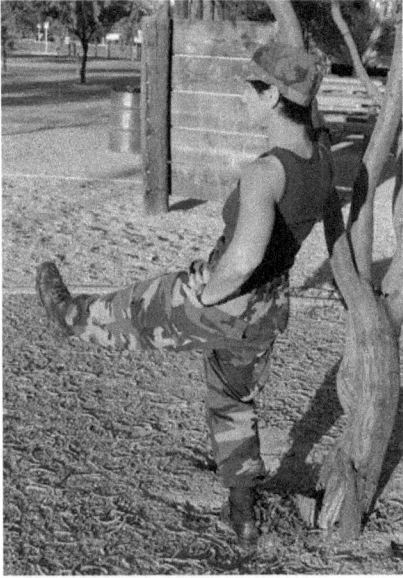

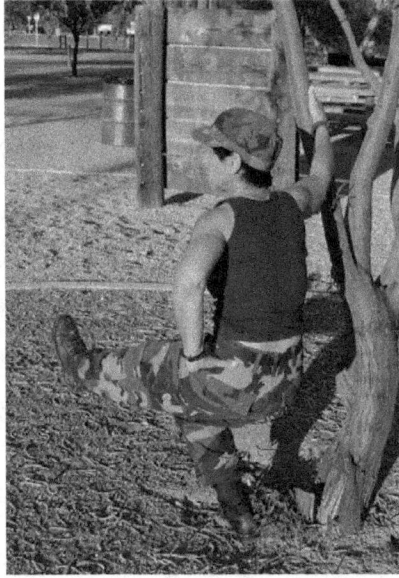

Heel Raise — You can do this on a curb or step or no, but be careful not to stretch too far and only perform if you are warmed up from walk or run or jumping jacks. Make certain you use a full range of motion. It won't take long to make this burn, and it works with weights too. Featured muscles used are gastrocnemius and soleus.

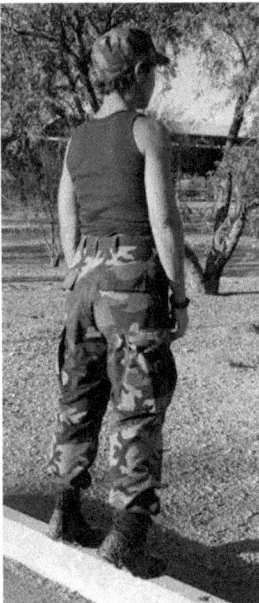

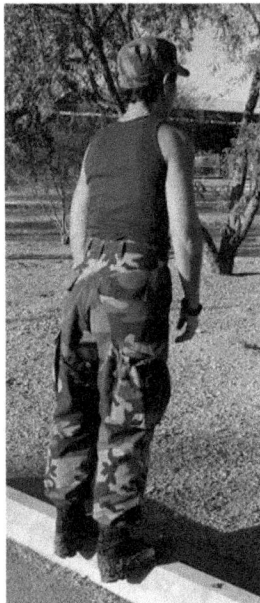

Walking Lunge — The lunge is a great leg exercise to develop shape and flexibility. Keep your chest up high and your stomach tight. Take a long step forward and drop your back knee toward the ground. Stand on your forward leg, bringing your feet together and repeat with the other leg. Make sure your knee never extends past your foot. Keep your shin vertical in other words. Muscles used: quadriceps, hams, and gluteus.

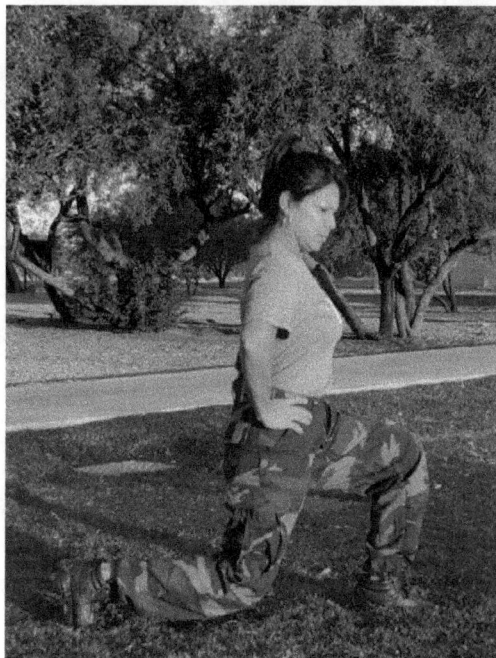

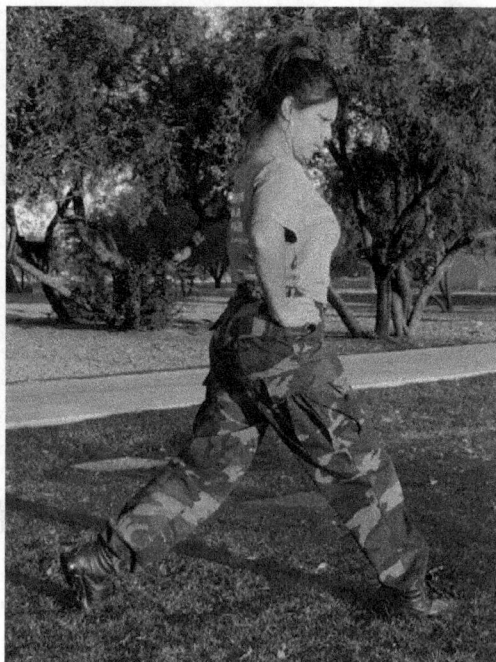

Name: Virginia Ellis
Age: 39
Buddy
How long in BCBC: 3 years
Occupation: Bookkeeper
Interests: Scuba Diving, Snowboarding, Quad Riding, Sand Duning,
& Hiking

Tender Shin Exercises — If you get shin splints from running or walking, here are two great exercises to build your shins. Stand on your heels for 10–15 seconds. Repeat a few times and even throughout the day to build your shins. Prior to walking and running, do the foot flex/stretch exercise 30–40 times each leg.

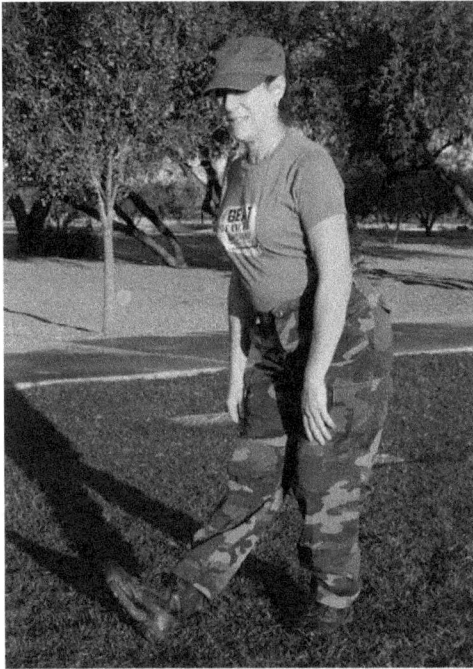

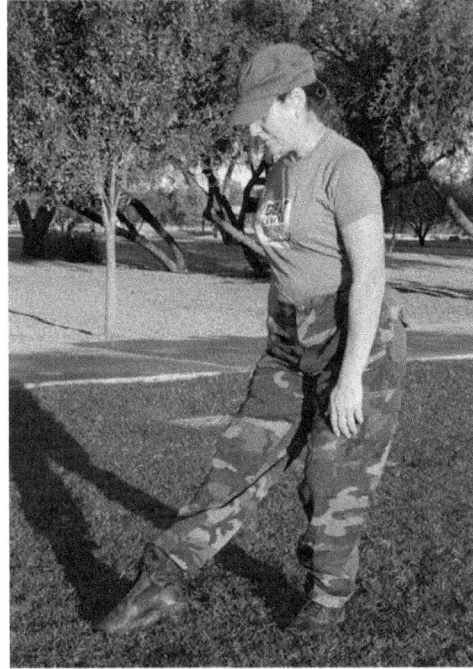

Name: Carol Margolis
Age: 56
Survivor: (type): Breast Cancer # years: 4 ½ years
How long in BCBC: 2 ¾ years
Occupation: Database Specialist
Something of Interest: Watershed management and Rainwater
Harvesting, sewing designs, gardening.

Dumbbell Exercises

Reverse Fly— With moderate weight dumbbells in each hand, bend over at the waist and slightly bend your knees. You want your back to be close to horizontal to the floor as you can. With your arms extended out to the side, lift your arms up and down as if you were a bird flying. Works upper back and stretches the chest and front shoulders.

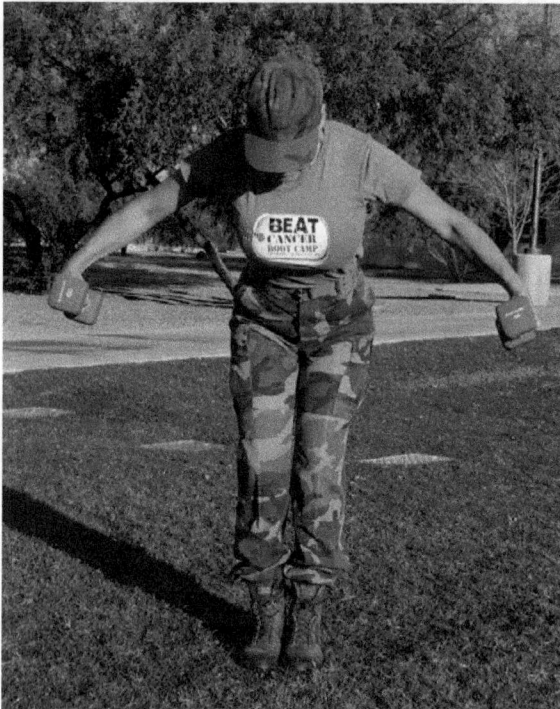

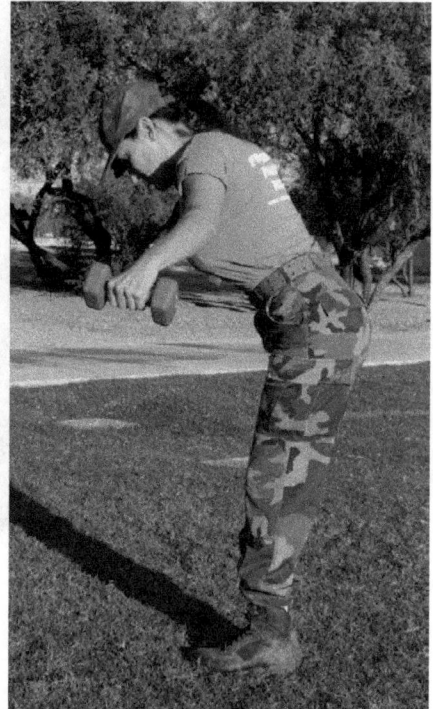

Name: Margo Susco
Age: 45
Buddy
# of Years in BCBC: 1 year
Occupation: Small Business Owner
Something of Interest: Love Classic Cars, Drag Racing,
Motorcycles, Big Band Music, and Ballroom Dancing

Bicep Curl — Place dumbbells or bar in hands with your palms facing upward. Use a complete range of motion and keep it smooth. Do not swing the weights. Nothing moves but your elbows. Muscles used: biceps (arms).

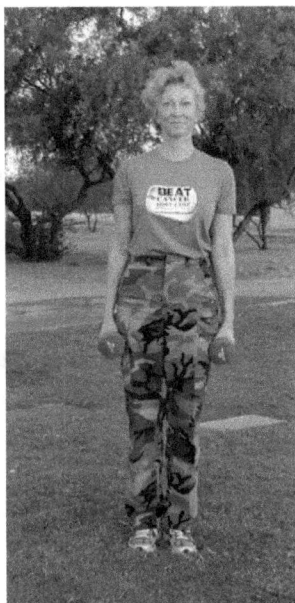

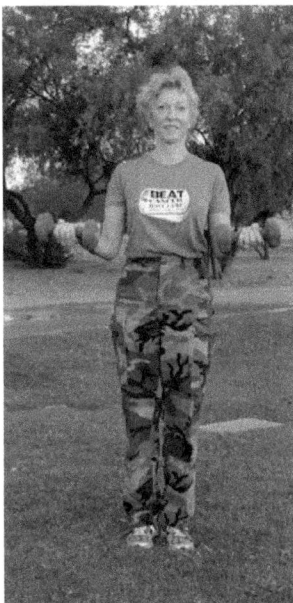

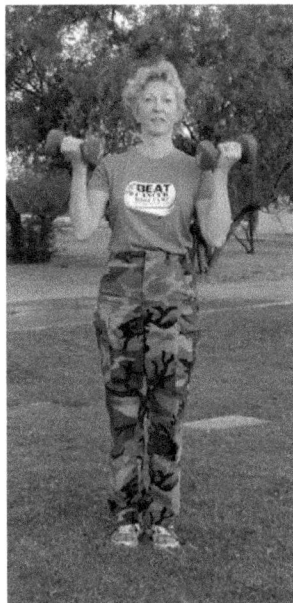

Bicep Curl — This is the same as a bicep curls except your palms are facing your hips. Alternate lifting each dumbbells like you were running "hip to lip." Use a complete range of motion and keep it smooth. Do not swing the weights.

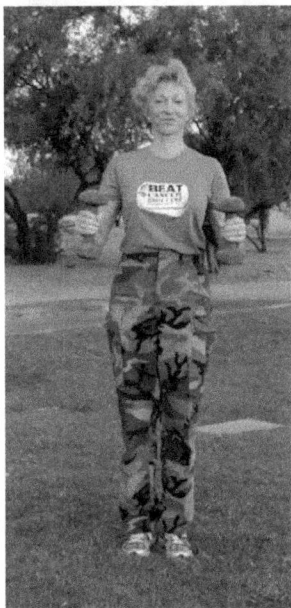

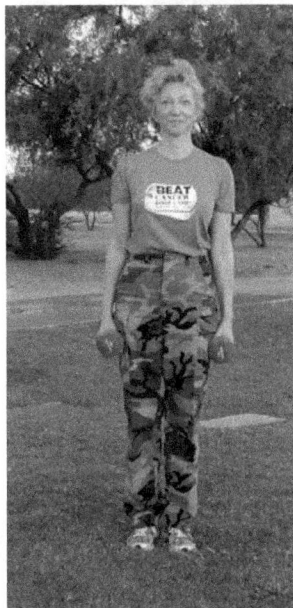

Name: Lana Holstein, MD
Age: 63
Survivor: (type): Colon Cancer
 # years: 8 years
How long in BCBC: 3 years
Occupation: Physician
Something of Interest:
Specialize in couples intimacy
and sexuality medicine. This
has been important for cancer
survivors as well.

Triceps extension — With weights in hands, bring your hands overhead and lower the weight toward the back of your neck. Make certain your elbows remain in one place through movement — next to your ears! Repeat!

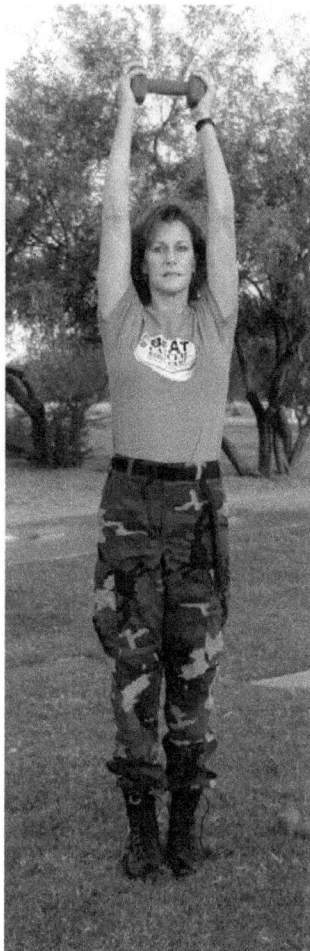

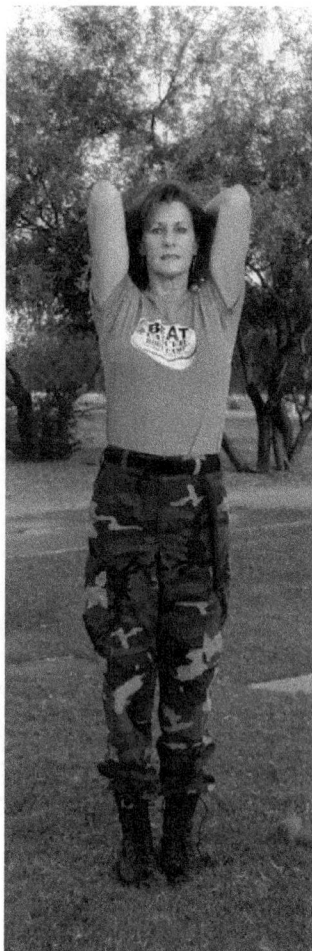

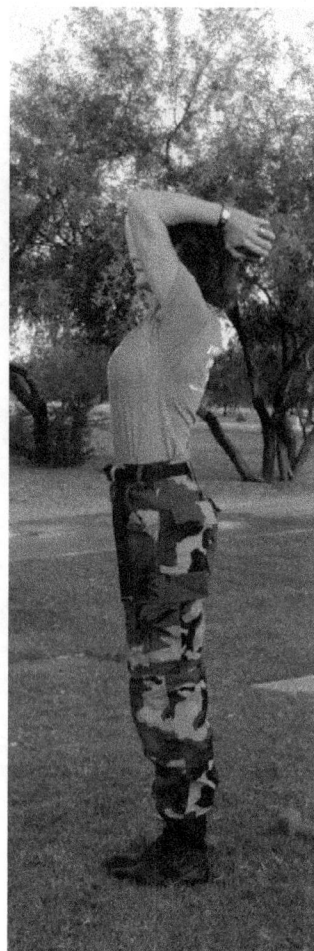

Name: Liz Almi
Age: 48
Survivor: (type): Breast # years: 4 years
How long in BCBC: 4 years
Occupation: Anesthesiologist, MD
Something of Interest: Married to Scott with boys Bryan & Alec.
Enjoy outdoor sports and family.

Bent Over Row — Bend over and support your lower back by placing your free hand on your outer thigh. Pull the dumbbell to your chest area as if you were starting a lawn mower. Muscles worked: Back, forearm grip, Bicep muscles.

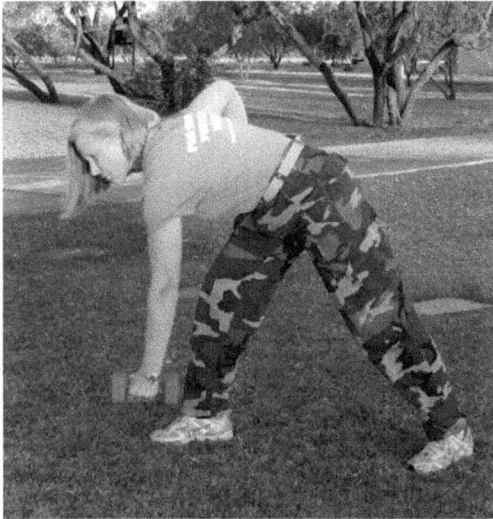

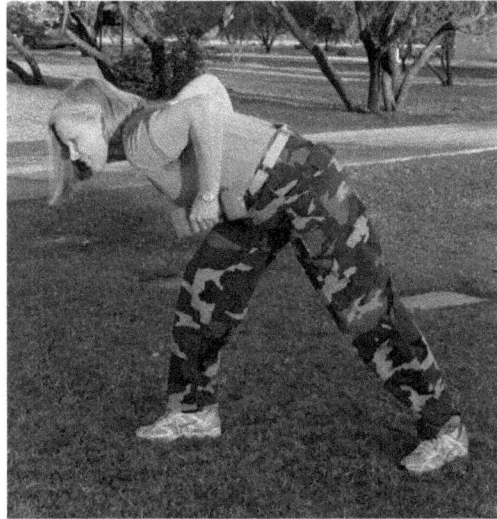

Name: Nancy Pearson
Age: 60
Survivor: (type): Breast # years: 7 years
How long in BCBC: 6 years
Occupation: Archaeologist/Researcher
Interest: I love xeriscape, gardening / houseplants. I enjoy cats with my partner of 24 years. I enjoy hiking, biking, exercising. I enjoy writing, and I love living!

Lightweight Shoulder Workout: (LWS)

When you see Shoulder Workout in a workout chart, refer to these six exercises.

Lateral Raise — This is a safe and effective shoulder exercise with light dumbbells (5 pound or under) or no weights. Using heavier dumbbells is not recommended for this exercise. Keep your knees slightly bent, shoulder back, and your chest high. Lift weights parallel to ground in a smooth controlled motion, keep your palms facing the ground. Follow the next SIX exercises without stopping.

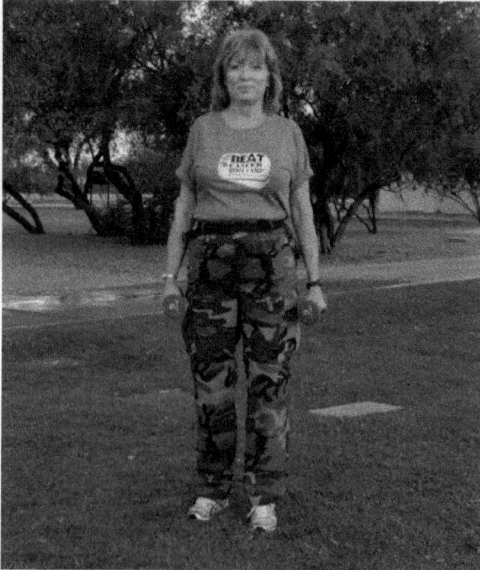

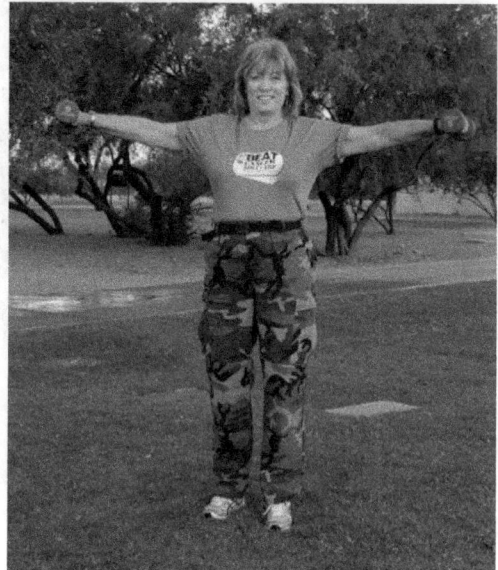

Name: Ginny Shaw
Age: 59
Survivor: (type): Breast/Colon # years: 8
How long in BCBC: 5 ½ years
Occupation: Retired
Something of Interest: I am an actress. I do accents as I taught in theatre for 30 years. I have a daughter.

Thumbs Up — After performing 10 regular lateral raises, do 10 lateral raises with your thumbs up, touching your hips with your palms facing away from you and raising your arms no higher than shoulder height.

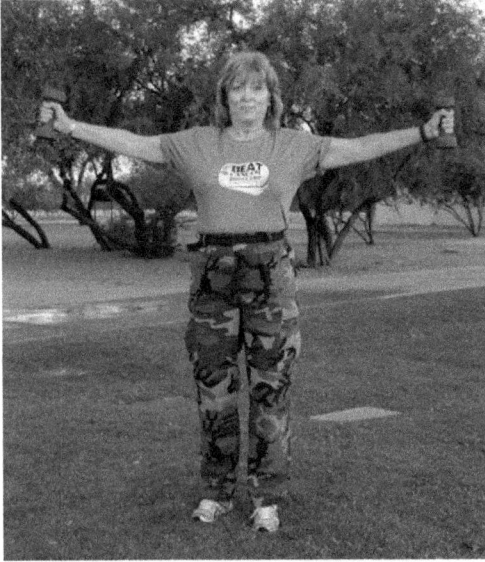

Thumbs Down — Continue with side lateral raises. As you lift your arms upward, keep your thumbs down up to shoulder height. Repeat for 10 times, always leading in the thumbs down direction.

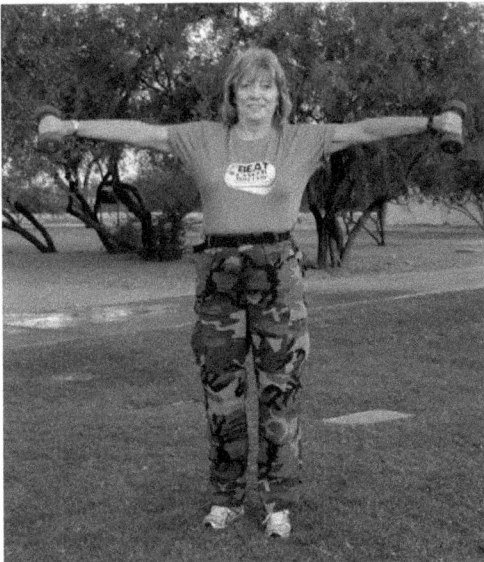

Front Raises (thumbs up) — Now for 10 more repetitions, time to work your front deltoids. Lift the dumbbells from your waist to shoulder height keeping your thumbs up.

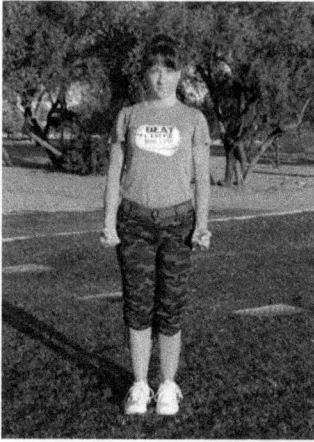

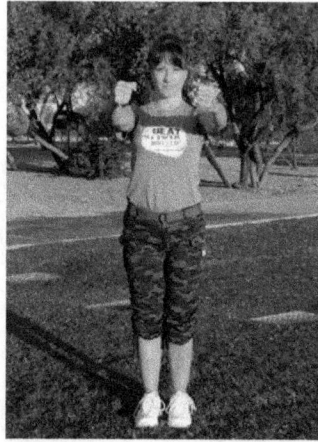

Cross Overs — With your palms facing away from you and arms relaxed in front of your hips, bring your arms up and over your head as if you were doing a jumping jack (without jumping). Cross your arms IN FRONT of your head and bring them back to your hips for 10 repetitions.

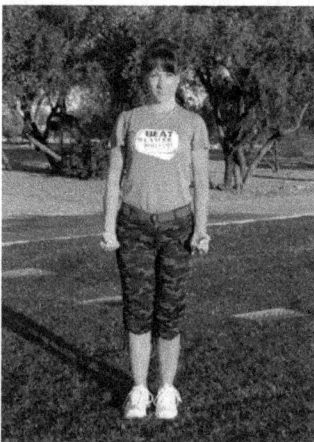

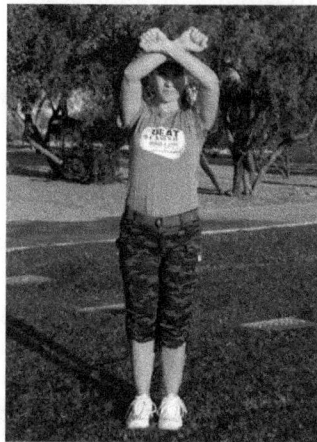

Name: Kathy Rozema
Age: 42
Survivor: Breast # years: 6 month
Occupation: Stay at home mom
Something of interest: I love G-d, my husband and my 5 children. Working out and shopping are my favorite things to do after traveling with my husband Terry.

Military Press — Place one foot ahead of the other as shown, with knees slightly bent to reduce strain on your lower back. Exhale as you push the weights over your head for 10 final repetitions in the mega-shoulder-pump workout. Slowly lower them to shoulder height and repeat. Muscles used are shoulders and triceps (back of arm).

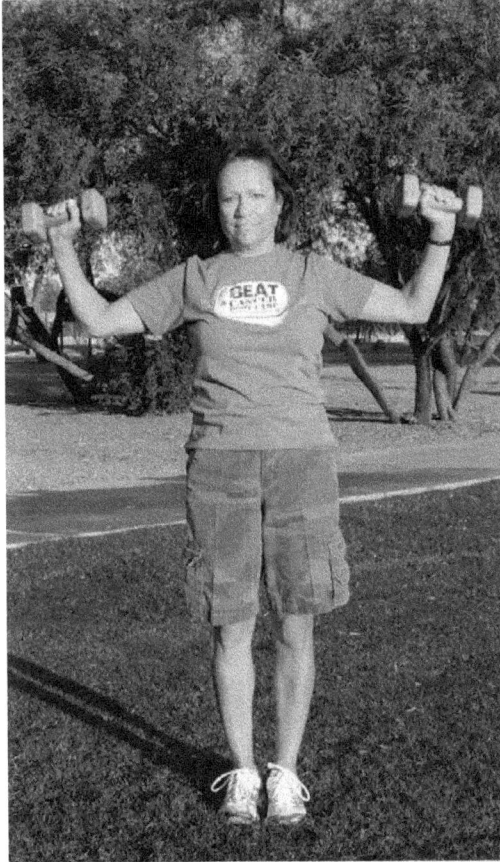

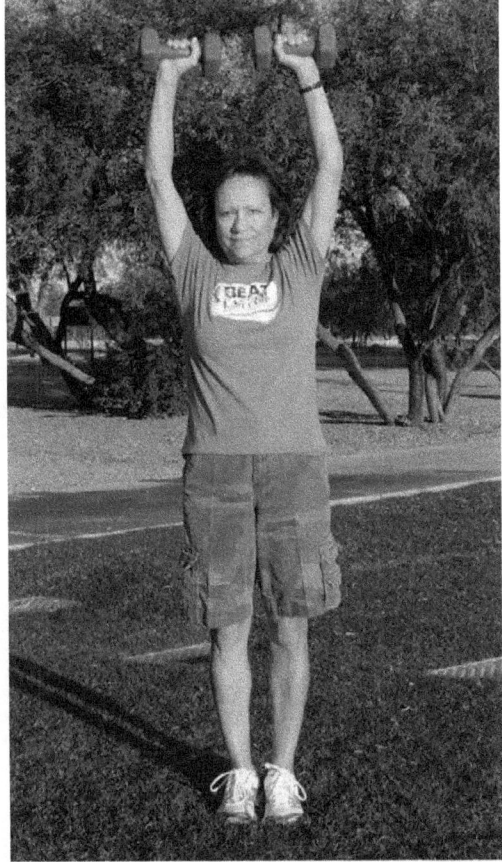

In conclusion, the Light Weight Shoulder workout consists of the six exercises done in back to back sequence without rest for 10 repetitions each:

Lateral Raises – 10 (palms down)
Lateral Raises – 10 (thumbs up)
Lateral Raises – 10 (thumbs down)
Front Raises – 10 (thumbs up)
Cross overs – 10 (palms facing away from you)
Military press – 10

Name: Pam Jameson
Age 54
Survivor : Breast # years: 3
How long in BCBC: 3 years
Something of interest: golf

Chest Fly/Press — Lie on your back with the dumbbells in your hands. Push the dumbbells straight up over your chest and repeat for 10-15 reps. Now with arms slightly bent, hold arms out as wide as you can until you touch your elbows to the ground and bring them back to the starting position with arms extended over your chest.

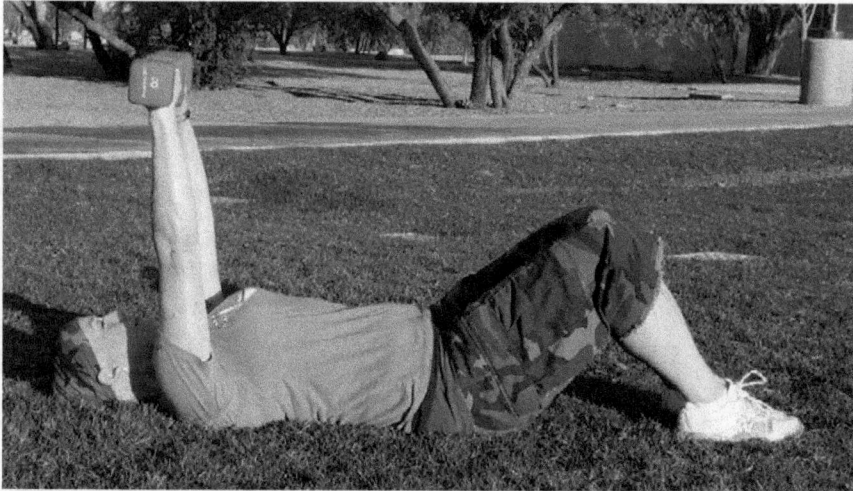

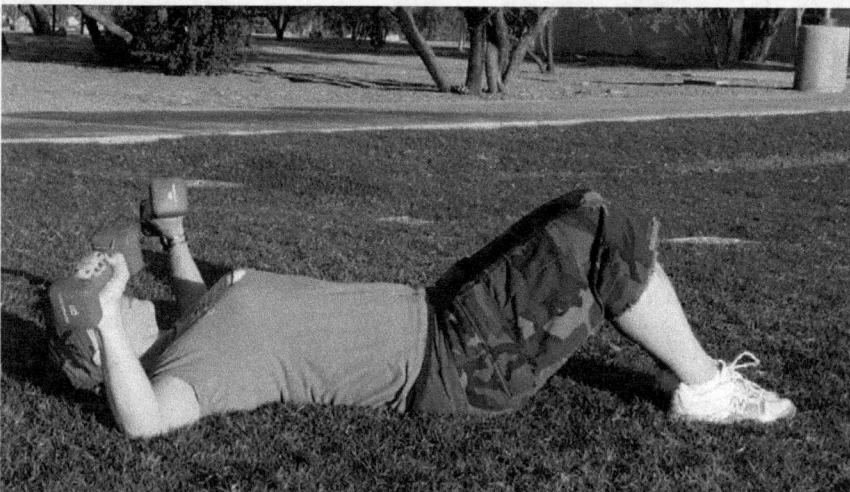

Name: Shannon Ortiz
Age: 37
Survivor: (type): Breast & Melanoma # years: 5 months/ 9years
How long in BCBC: 6 months
Occupation: Sales Supervisor
Something of Interest: Spending time with or chasing after my 3 young kids and husband! The kid's sports are a lot of fun for us right now!

Tricep Dips — Using a bench, chair, or curb, sit on edge with hands just outside your hips on the object you are sitting on. Lower yourself until you reach a 90 degree angle in the elbows or until your rump touches the floor (whichever comes first). Lift yourself back to the starting position in your seat.

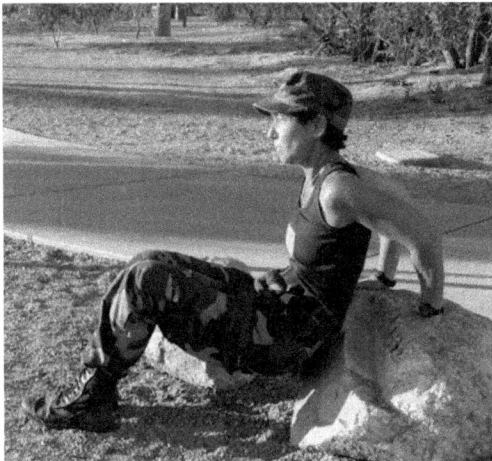

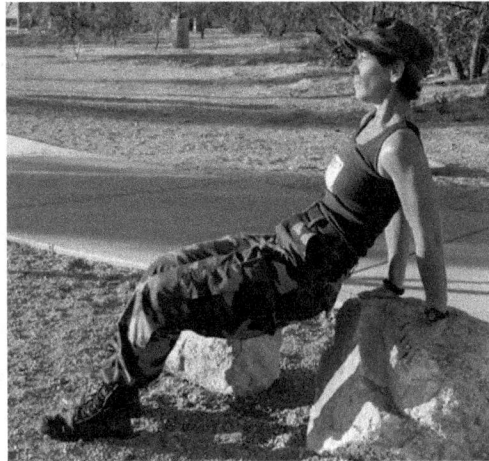

Abdominals – The Crunch Cycle

Defined *Crunch cycle — 10–20 of each exercise:
Regular Crunch — shoulders blades off floor
Reverse Crunch — hips off floor
Double Crunch - both hips/shoulders off floor at the same time
Left crunches — 20
Right crunches — 20 (elbow toward opposite knees)
Plank pose 30 seconds
Stretch stomach

The following exercises are part of the "Crunch Cycle" that you will see in the workout charts. You will try to perform ALL crunches below for the amount of reps listed in the workout chart. For instance, if you see Crunch Cycle – 10 – that means you will do all exercises below for 10 reps each. Resting with stomach stretches is allowed too. Follow a crunch cycle with a few lower back plank poses as well for torso balance.

When you exercise your stomach muscles, make sure to exercise and stretch your back also. The stomach and lower back muscles are opposing muscle groups and if one is much stronger than the other, then you can injure the weaker muscle group easily, usually the lower back.

Regular Crunch — Lie on your back with your feet and knees in the air with the knees bent. Cross your hands over your chest and bring your elbows to your knees by flexing your stomach. Keep your feet on the floor if your lower back is weak or previously injured.

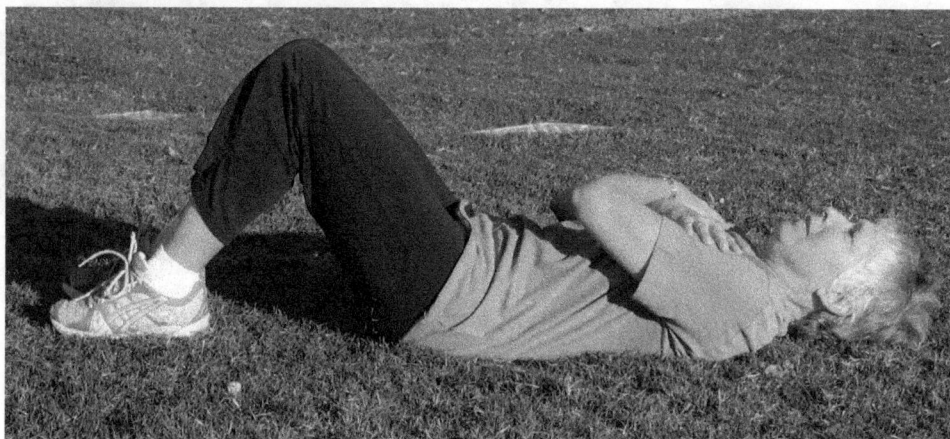

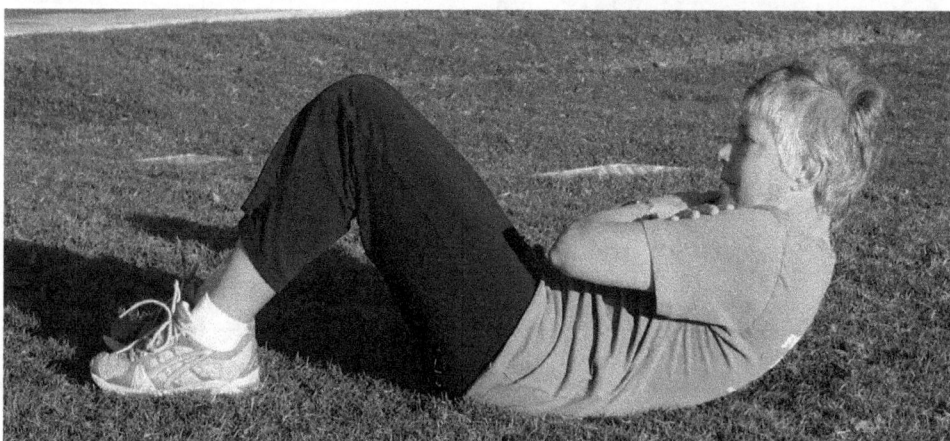

Name: Laura Gibson
Age: 58
Survivor: (type): breast # years: 1 year
How long in BCBC: 1 year
Occupation: Jewelry Designer
Something of Interest: Cycling, kayaking

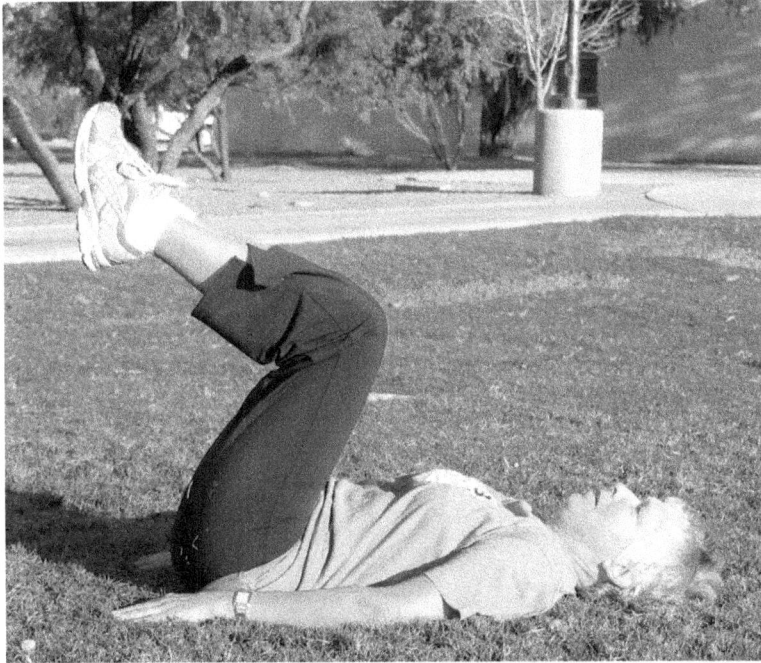

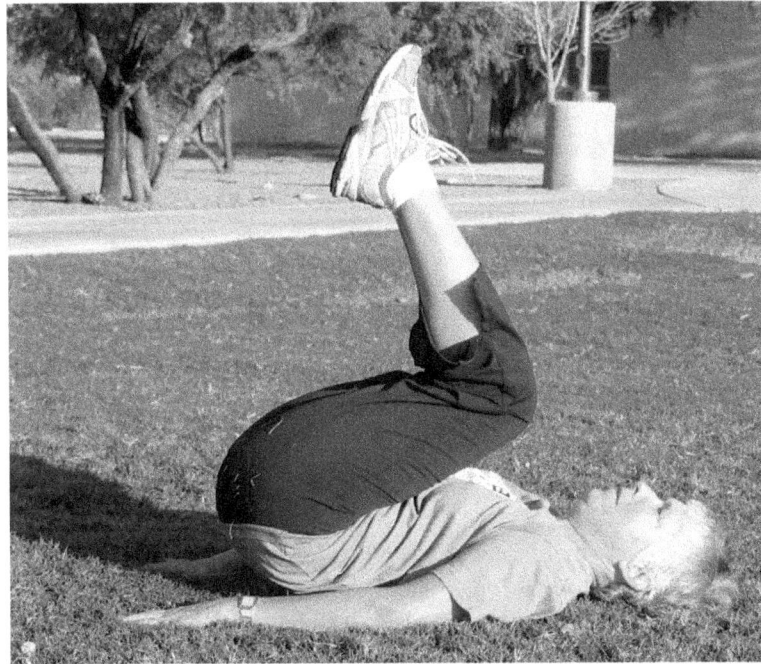

Right Elbow to Left Knee — Cross your left leg over your right leg. Flex your stomach and twist to bring your right elbow to your left knee.

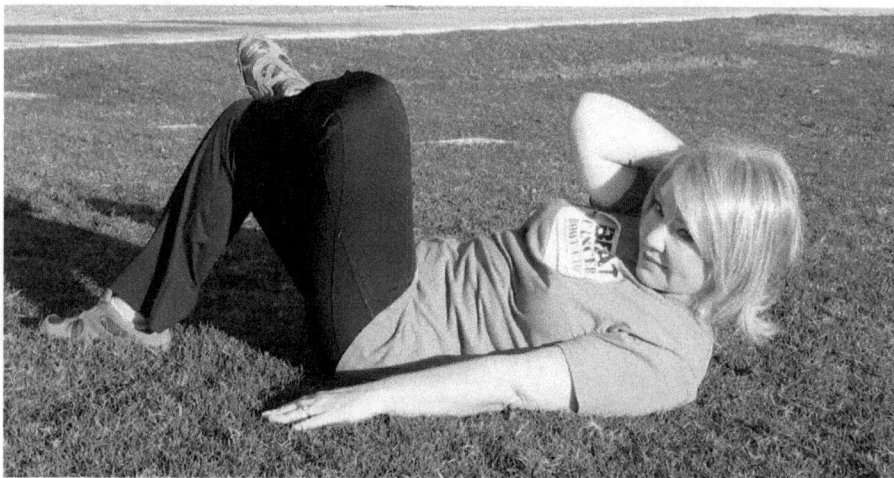

Left Elbow to Right Knee — Cross your right leg over your leg. Flex your stomach and twist to bring your left elbow to your right knee.

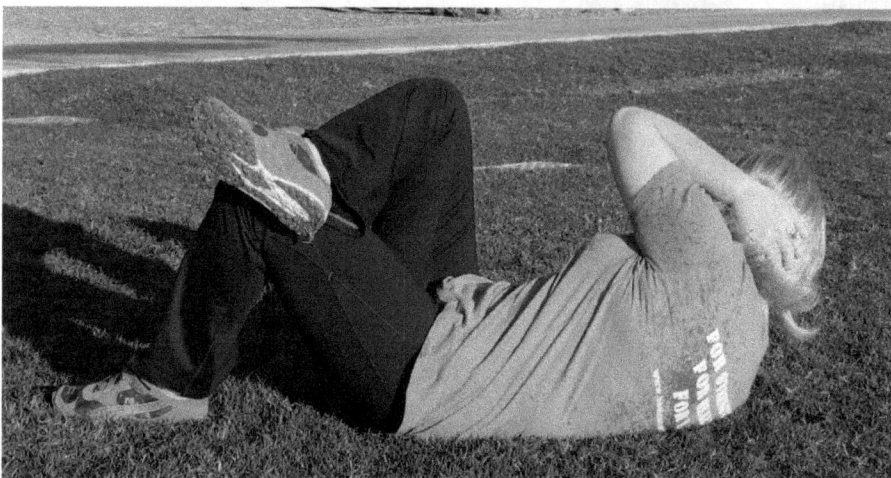

Name: Jan Minas
Age: 58
Survivor: (type): Breast Cancer # years: 1 ½ years
Number of Years in BCBC: 1 year plus
Occupation: Retired Bed & Breakfast Owner & Home Economics Teacher
Something of Interest: Live in the mountains at the Saguaro National Park Monument West. I love my husband, children, dogs and boot camp!

Double Crunch (Legs up) — Lie on your back with your feet in the air. Lift your head/shoulders off the floor toward your knees by flexing your stomach AND lift your hips off the floor as if you were doing a reverse crunch at the same time. This is two crunches in one movement.

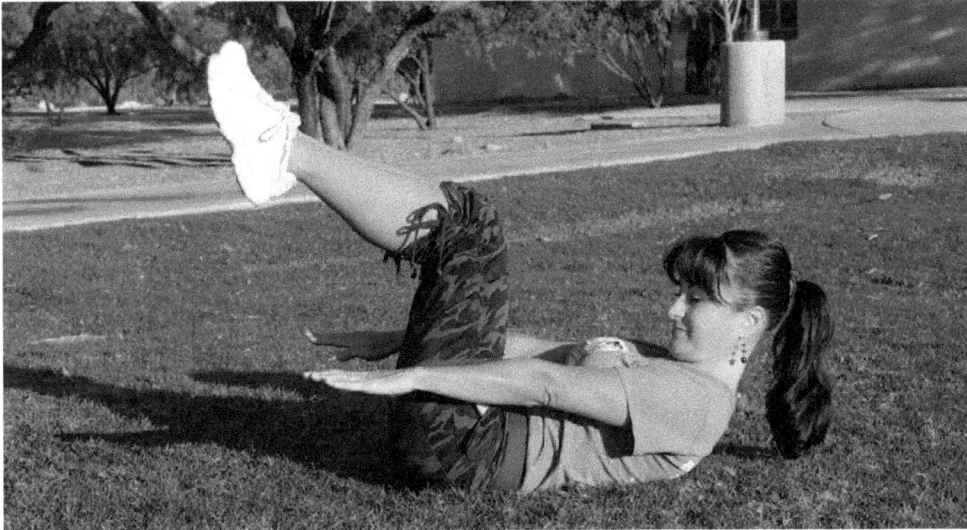

Bicycle Crunches — Peddle your legs back and forth as shown while doing left and right crunches. This is a tough one, so if your back hurts, stop and skip these until your back is stronger.

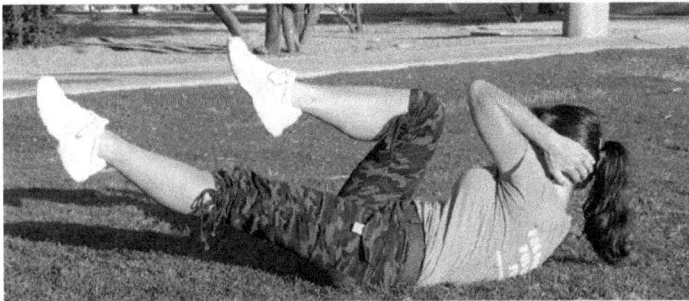

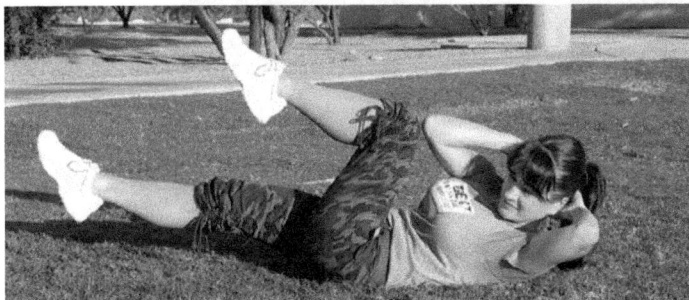

Name: Kathy Rozema
Age: 42
Survivor: (type): breast
 # years: 6 months
Occupation: Mom
How long in BCBC:
6 months
Something of Interest: I love God, my husband and my 5 children. Working out and shopping are my favorite things to do after travelling with my husband Terry.

Lower Back/Abs Exercise Section

Plank Pose — Keep your back straight and abs tight while placing your elbows and toes on the floor and holding for as long as you can. Build up to 1min. Advanced is 3–5min.

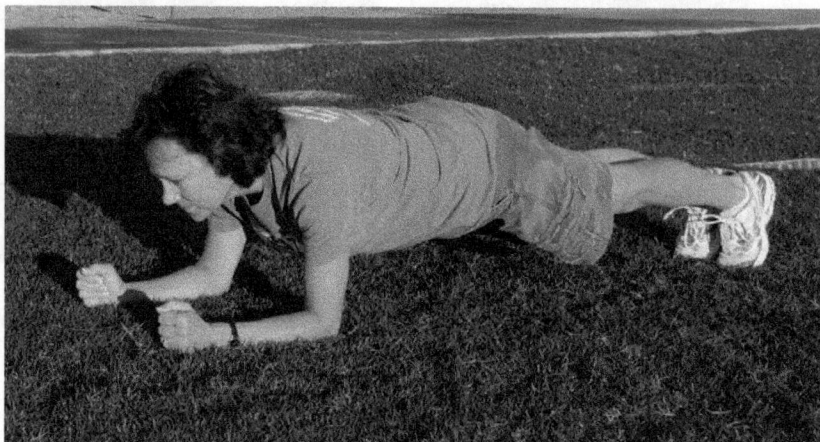

Plank Pose advanced — **Pushup** — **Up Position** — Tighten abs and keep your back straight. If shoulders bother you or arms are not built up, do this same exercise on your elbows where only your elbows and toes are touching.

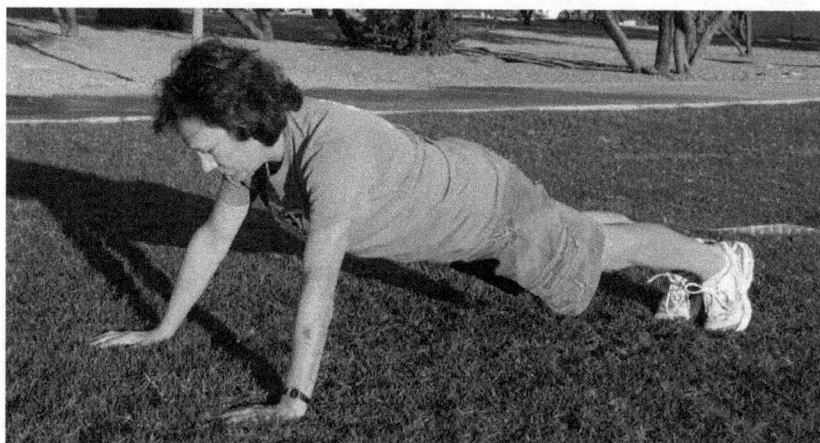

Name: Pam Jameson
Age 54
Survivor : Breast # years: 3
How long in BCBC: 3 years
Something of interest: golf

As you know, the lower back one of the most commonly injured areas of the body. Many lower back problems stem from inactivity, lack of flexibility, improper lifting of heavy objects, as well as hip and leg muscle instability. Stretching and exercising your lower back, hips, and legs will help prevent some of those injuries.

Lower Back Exercise (Swimmers) — Lie on your stomach and lift your feet and knees off the floor by flutter kicking repeatedly as if you were swimming freestyle. Build up to one minute, or hold feet still but off the floor to fill out the minute.

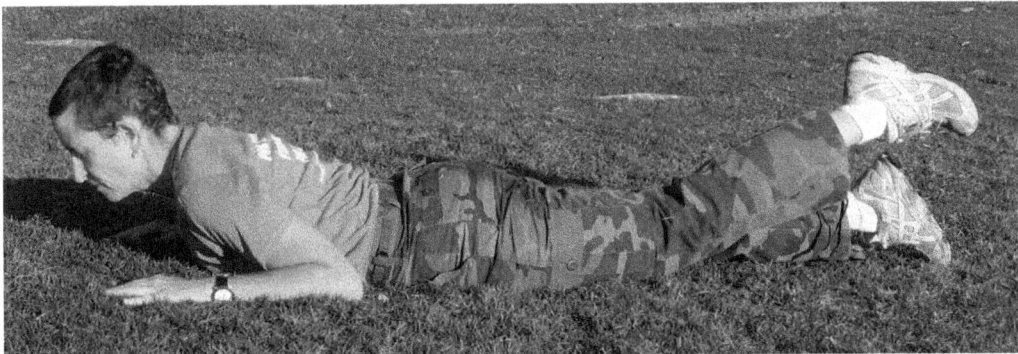

Name: Shawn Mulligan
Age: 47
Survivor: (type): breast # years: 9 months
How long in BCBC: 4 months
Occupation: Nurse
Something of Interest: Cycled 250 miles with my family friends and our small kids- along the Erie Canal in NY!

Upper Back exercise #1 (Reverse Pushups) — Lie on your stomach in the down pushup position. Lift your hands off the floor instead of pushing the floor. This will strengthen your upper back muscles that oppose the chest muscles. Rear deltoids and rhomboids are the muscles used.

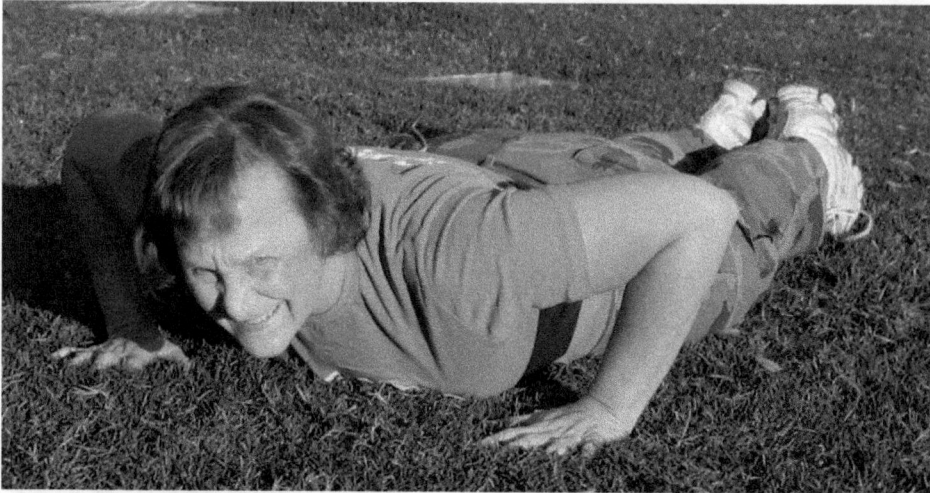

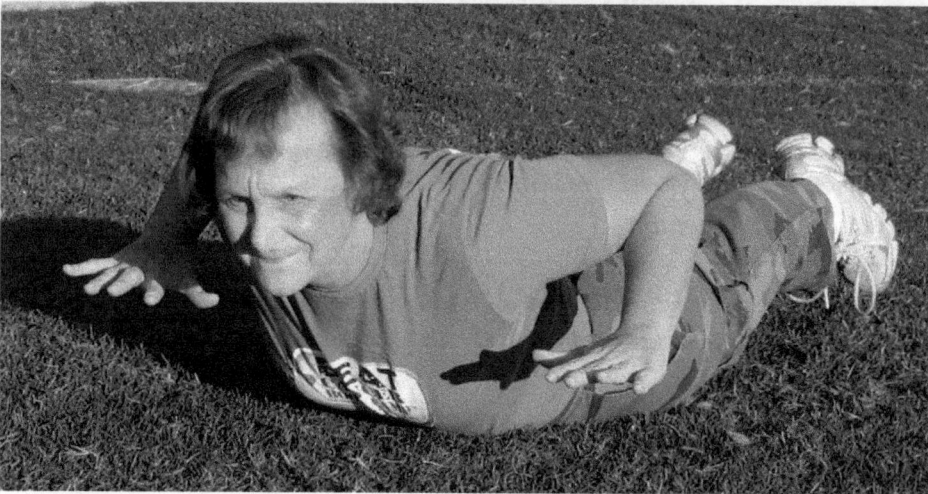

Name: Sarah Hondrum
Age: 52
Survivor: (type): Breast # years: 1 year
How long in BCBC: 17 months
Occupation: Nurse
Something of Interest: When I was diagnosed, I was put to work on the oncology floor of the hospital in discharge. When my hair fell out, I had instant credibility.

Upper Back #2 - Arm Haulers — Lie on your stomach with your arms spread to the height of your shoulders. Lift both arms off the floor and raise them over your head like you were doing a jumping jack. Repeat for 10-15 repetitions, mimicking a horizontal jumping jack (although your feet do not move).

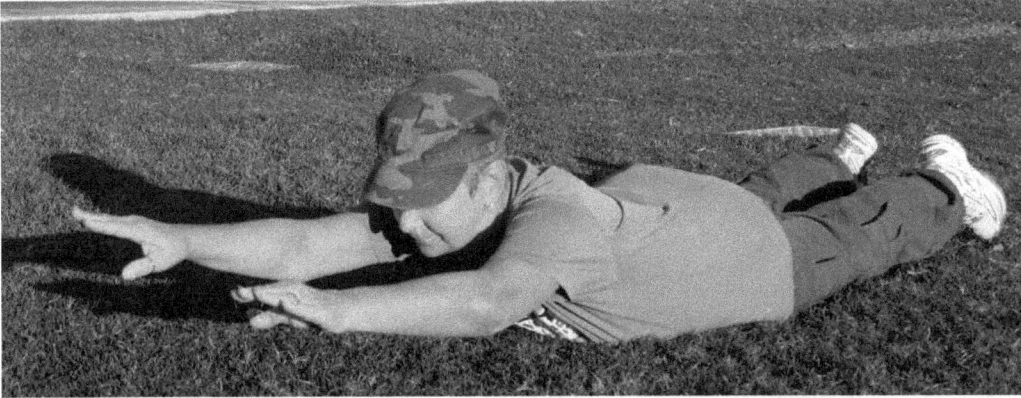

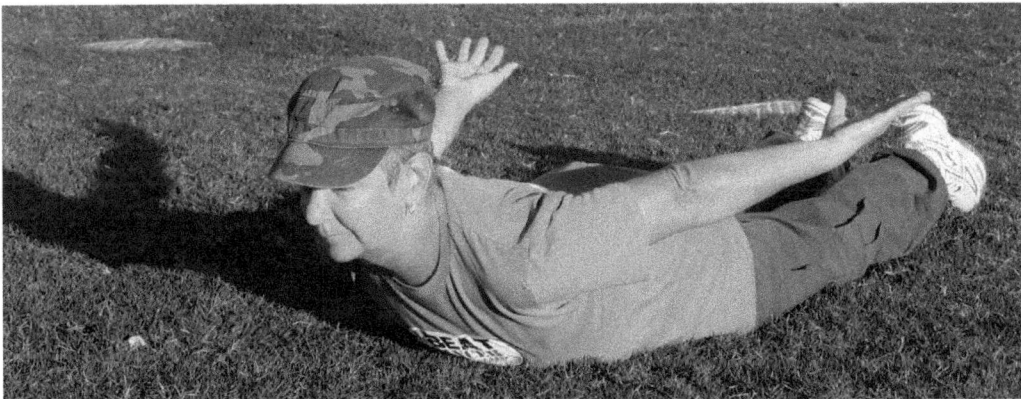

Name: Carol Cueto
Age: 62
Survivor: (type): Breast # years: I year
How long in BCBC: 3 months
Occupation: Retired
Something of Interest: My husband and I love to ride our tandem and go to Starbuck's for coffee.

Advanced Abdominal Exercises:

Do not try these if you are a beginner! These exercises are a risk for weak or injured backs. If you cannot do the swimmer exercises for a minute, do not attempt these exercises.

To reduce strain on the lower back, lift your butt off the ground about an inch and place your hands underneath your butt bone. Lay one hand on top of the other to get a higher lift of the butt, thus taking some of the strain off the lower back. Keep your knees straight and do these exercises at a full range of motion of your hips (legs 6 inches off the floor to vertical).

Situps — Lie on your back with your arms crossed over your chest, keeping your knees slightly bent. Raise your upper body off the floor by contracting your abdominal muscles. Touch your elbows to your thighs and repeat. If you are going Army - you have to place your hands behind your head.

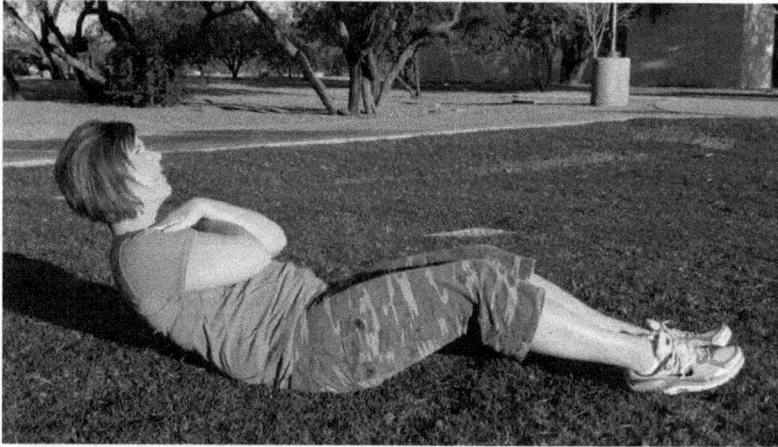

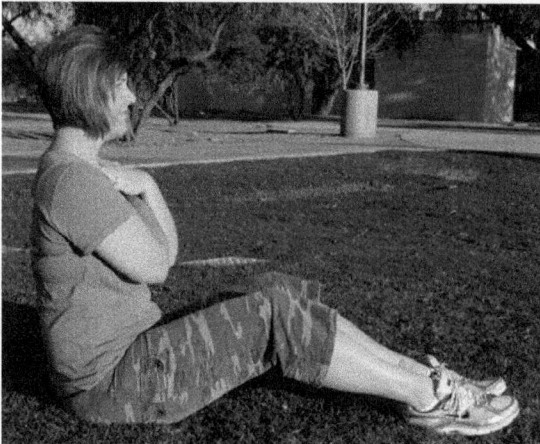

Cross Situps (L/R Situps) — Lie on your back with your knees bent and feet flat on the floor. Raise your upper body off the floor but add a slight twist and touch your left elbow to your right knee and return your back to the floor. Alternate and touch your right elbow to your left knee and repeat the sequence.

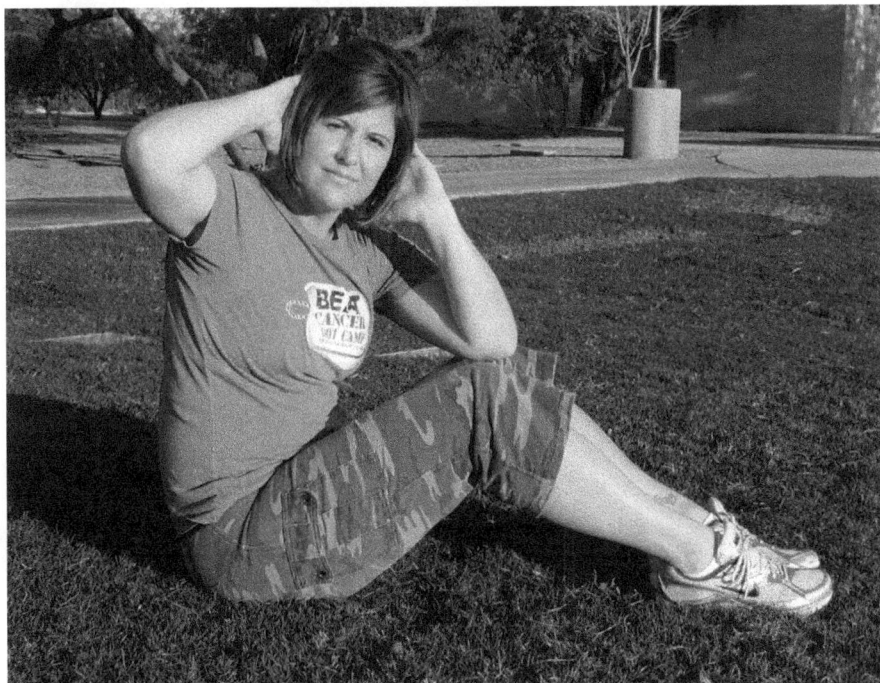

Name: Erin Resnick Age: 36
How long in BCBC: 6 months
Occupation: Mom
Something of Interest: I love spending time with friends and family.
Boot camp is fun and challenging! I look forward to it!

Flutter Kicks — Place your hands under your hips. Lift your legs 6 inches off the floor and begin walking, raising each leg approximately 36 inches off the ground. Keep your legs straight and moving. This is a four-count exercise.

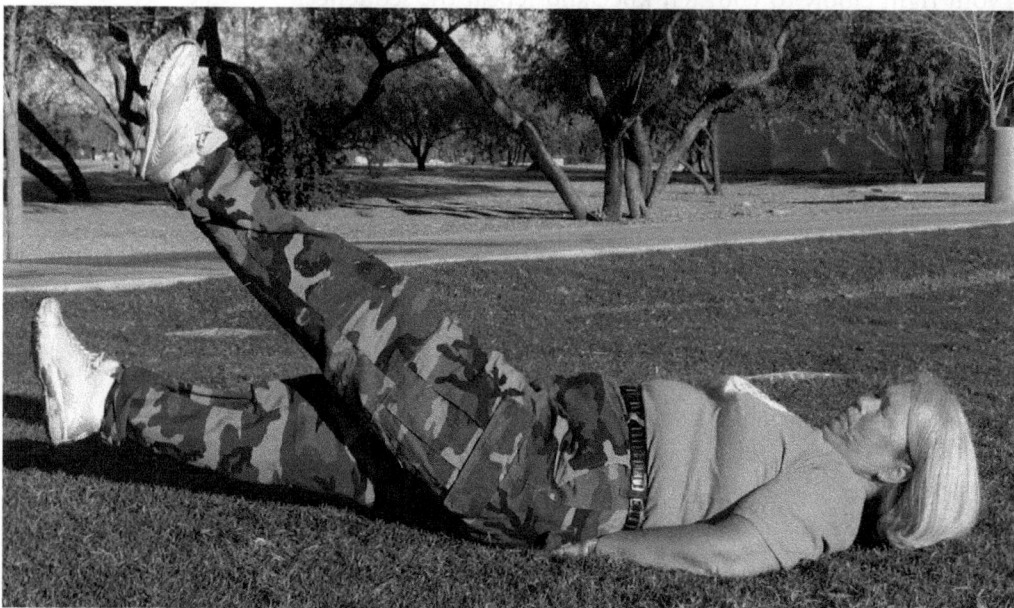

Name: Donna Shaw
Age: 61
Survivor: (type): Breast # years: 4
Occupation: Retired
Something of Interest: Golf

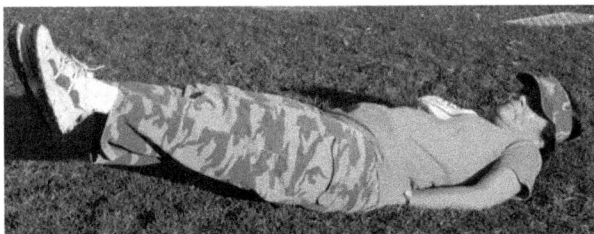

Leg Levers — Lift your feet 6 inches off the floor. Raising both legs approximately 36 inches off the ground, keep your legs straight and off the floor until you complete the specified number of repetitions.

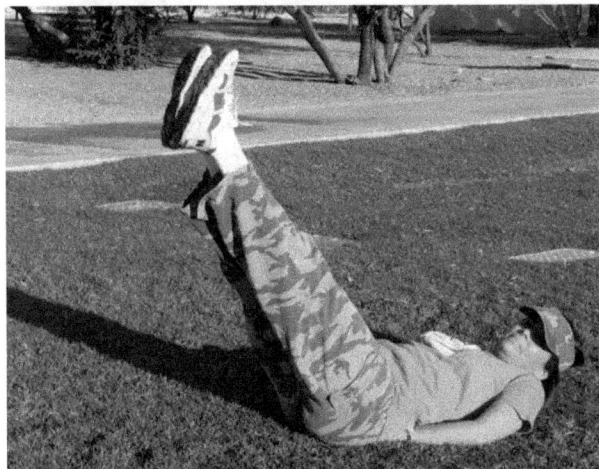

Scissors — Lie on your back. Lift your feet 6 inches off the floor. Open and close both legs approximately 36 inches apart, keep your legs straight and off the floor until you do the specified number of repetitions.

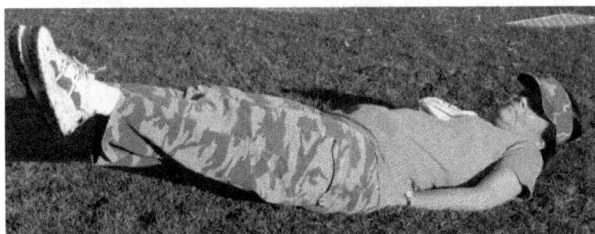

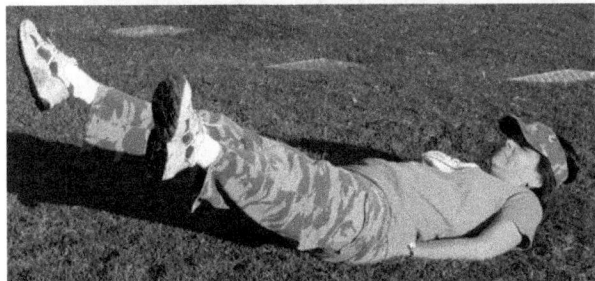

Name: Natalie DeWeese
Age: 51
Buddy
Number of Years in BCBC:
4 years
Occupation: Marketing
Manager
Something of Interest: I love
to travel and cook. I enjoy
spending time with my
husband and children

Aomic Situps — Lift your feet 6 inches off the floor as if you were doing a leg lever. Pull your knees toward your chest while simultaneously lifting your upper body off the floor. This is a mix between the situp and the leg lever.

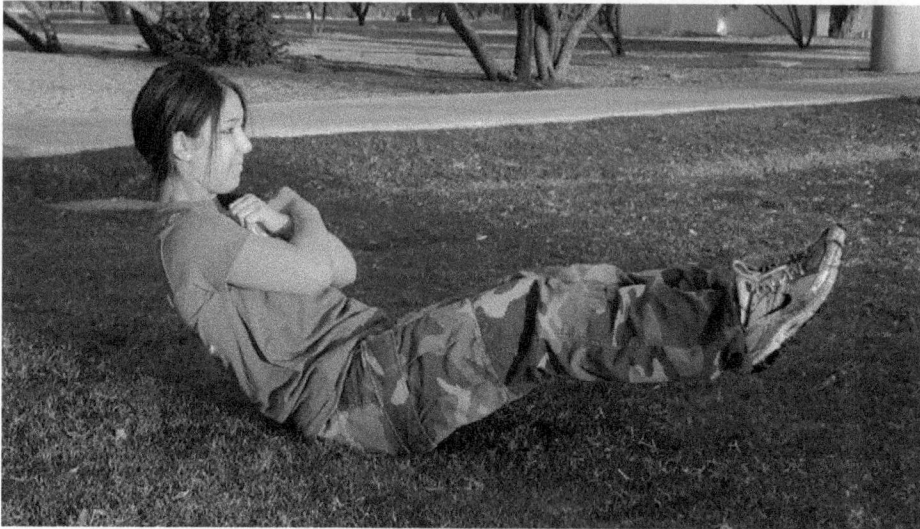

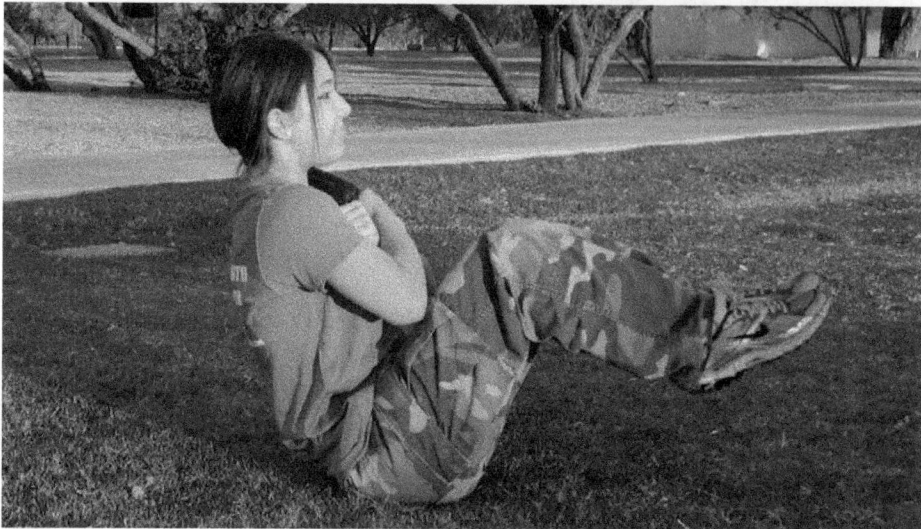

Name: Marlee Kellman
Age: 15
Buddy
How long in BCBC: 5 years
Occupation: Student
Something of Interest: Volleyball, spending time with friends, working with kids.

Hip Rolls — Lie flat on your back with your knees in the air as in the middle picture below. Keep your shoulders on the floor, rotate your hips and legs to the left and right as shown below.

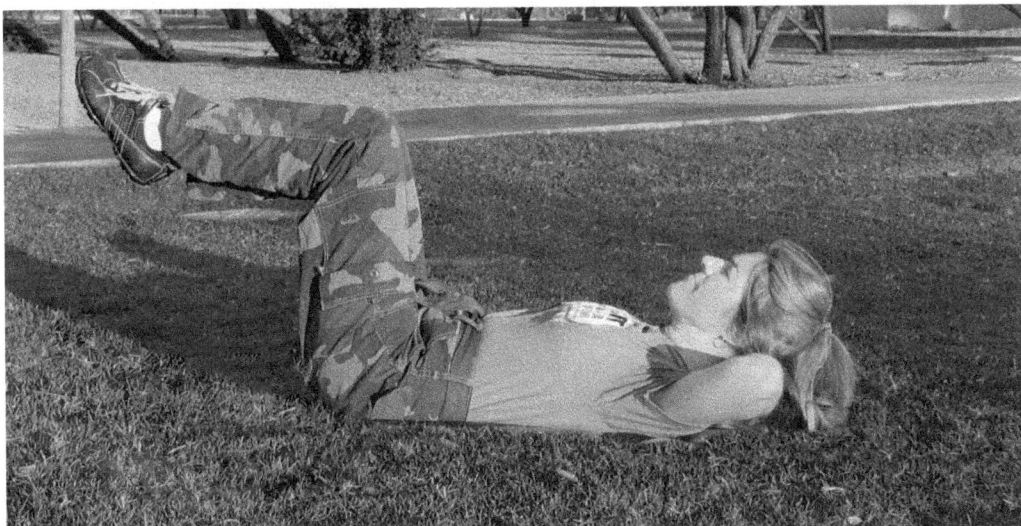

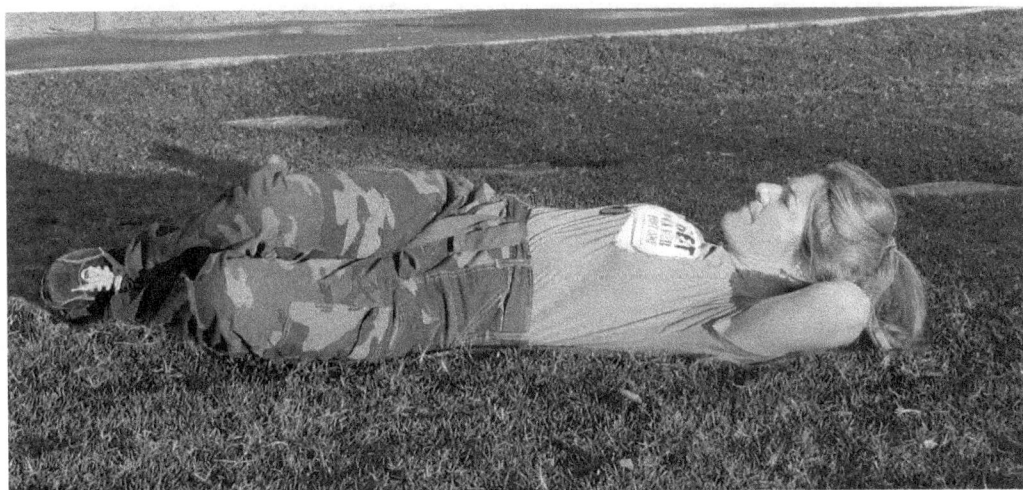

Name: Colleen Mathis
Age: 43
Survivor: (type): Breast # years: 3 years
How long in BCBC: 2 years
Occupation: Healthcare Administrator
Something of Interest: Arizona History, Radio, Travel, Music, & Cooking

Donkey Kicks — In the all-fours position, lift right leg as high as you can and bring the knee back to the floor. Repeat as required (great for hip stretch and pelvic girdle development).

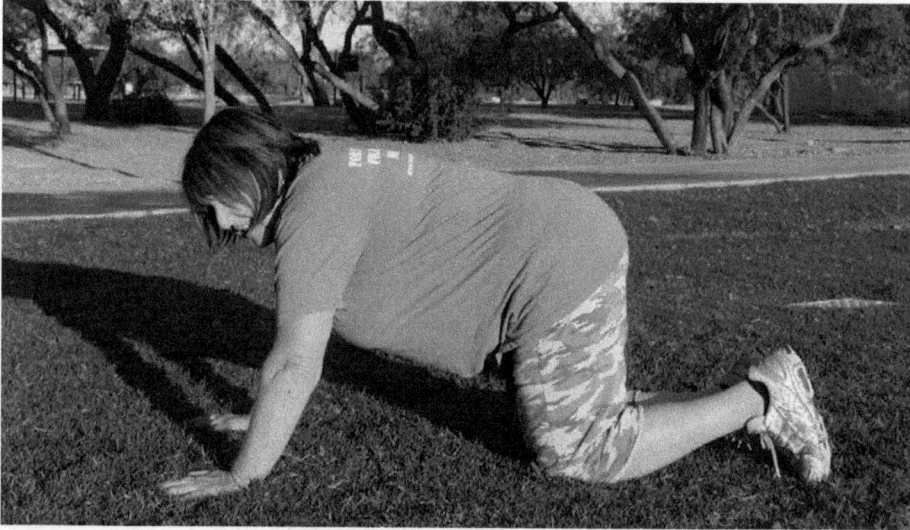

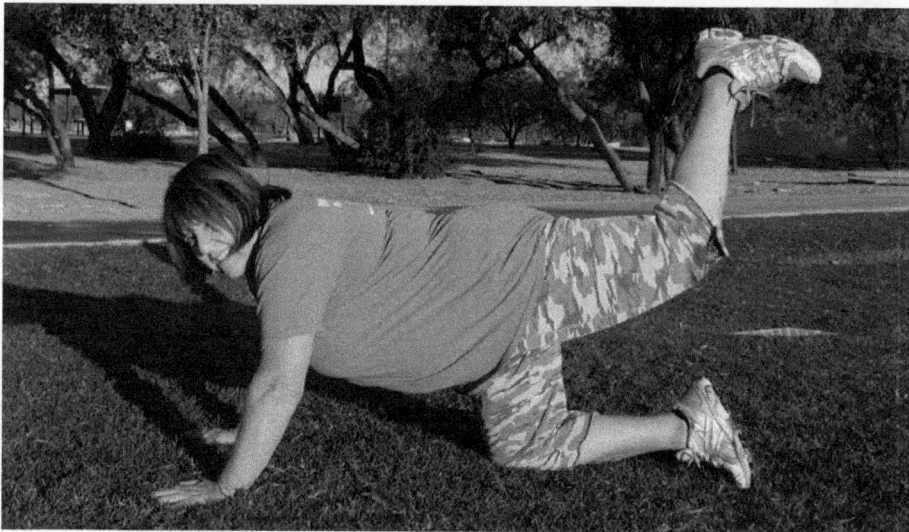

Name: Soozie Hazan
Age: 64
Survivor: (type): Breast # years: 6 ½
How long in BCBC: 6 years
Occupation: Faculty at Pima Community College
Something of Interest: I enjoy teaching and I have done it for over 30 years in different schools. My hobby is gardening!

Dirty Dogs — In the all-fours position again, lift your right leg from the hip as shown and repeat this cycle for suggested repetitions.

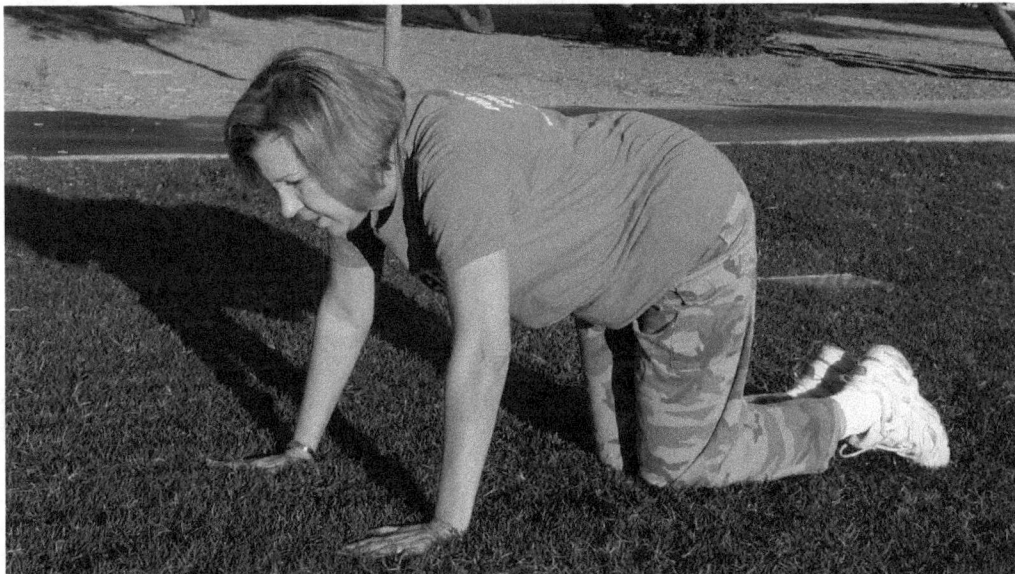

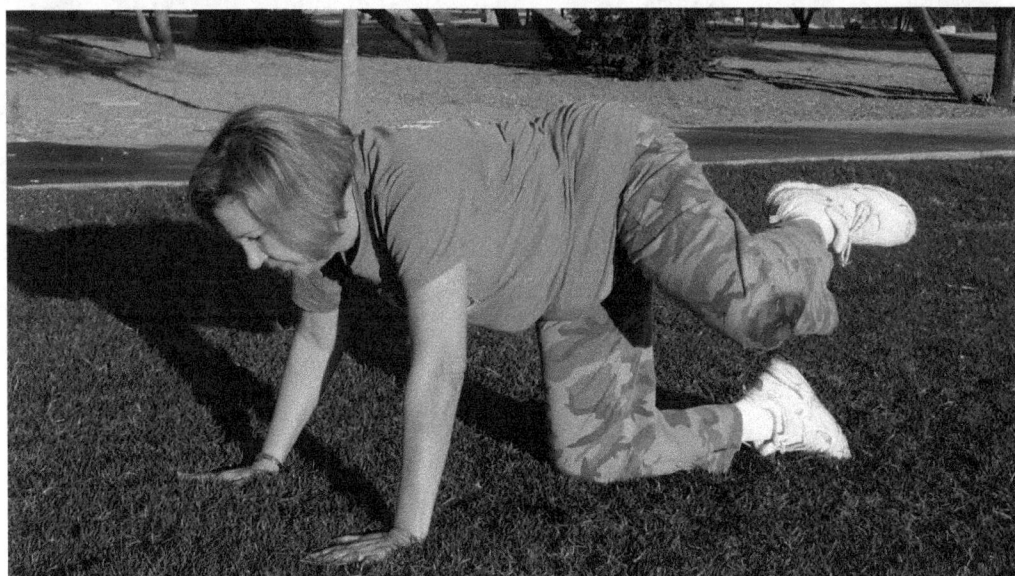

Name: Arlene Kutoroff Age: 60
Survivor: (type): Breast # years: 3 years
How long in BCBC: 2 ½ years
Occupation: Retired School Counselor
Something of Interest: Wine-tasting

Bear Crawls — Walk like a bear on all fours. This gets tough after a minute.

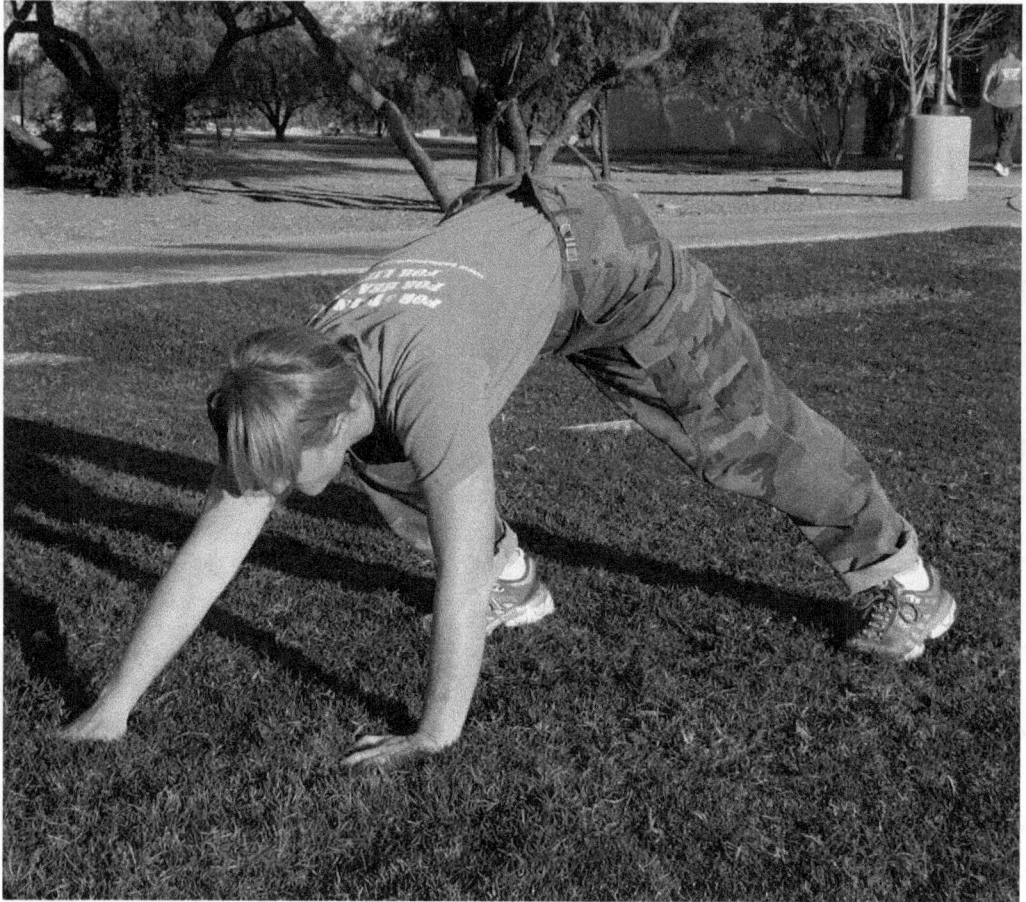

Name: Cathy Pensak
Age: 47
Buddy
How long in BCBC: 4 months
Occupation: Healthcare Administrator
Something of Interest: Working mother, love anything that will take me outdoors.
Running, biking, hiking. My mother is a cancer survivor.

Pushups
Advanced PT (Body weight exercises)

Regular Pushups — Lie on the ground with your hands placed flat next to your chest. Your hands should be about shoulder width apart. Push yourself up by straightening your arms and keeping your back straight. Look forward as you perform this exercise. This exercise will build and firm your shoulders, arms, and chest. See other variations for easier ways to perform this exercise.
Show them how it is done Sarge!

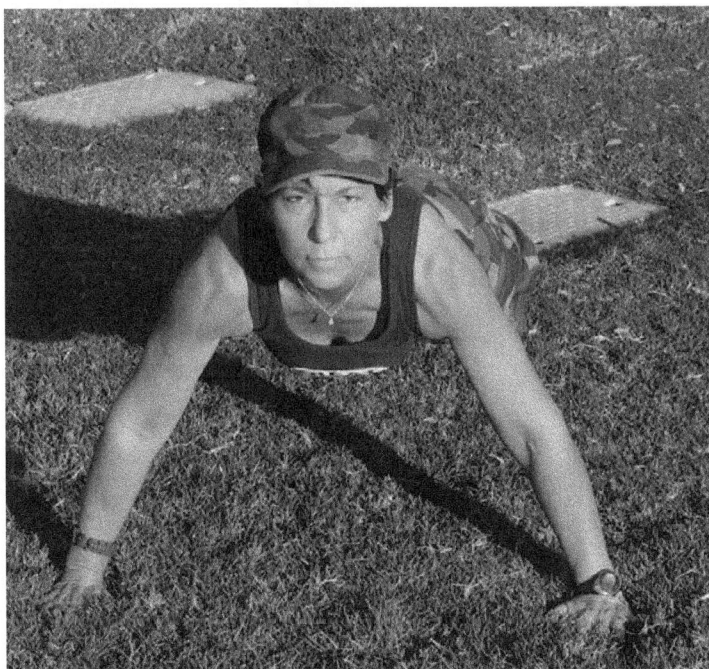

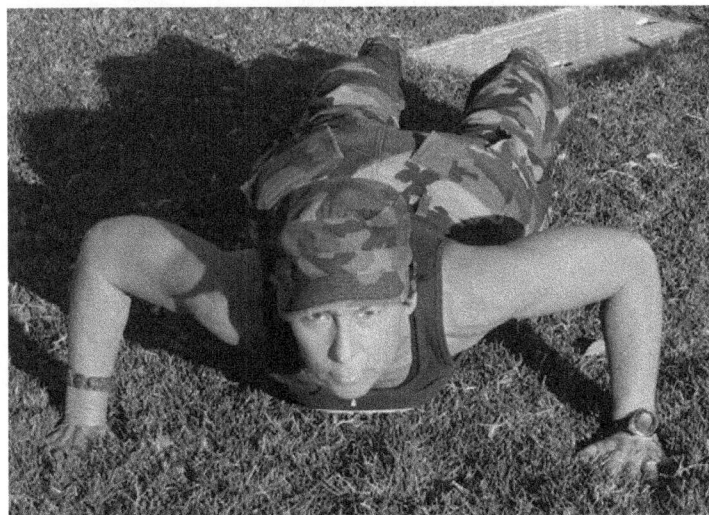

Easier Version — You can always start the pushup on your knees but you can also use a sturdy piece of furniture or equipment.

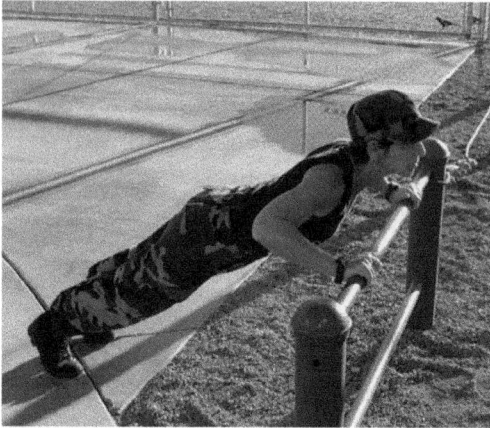

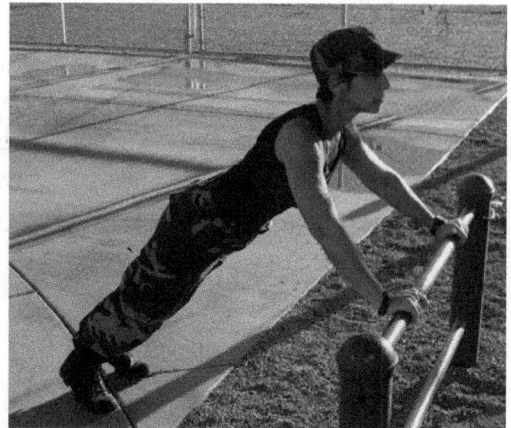

Wide Pushups — From the same position as the previous push-up, place your hands about six to twelve inches away from your chest. Your hands should be greater than shoulder width apart. The slight change of the arm distance changes the focus of what muscle are exercised. Now you are building the chest more than your arms and shoulders.

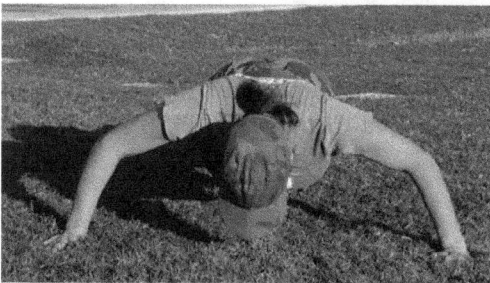

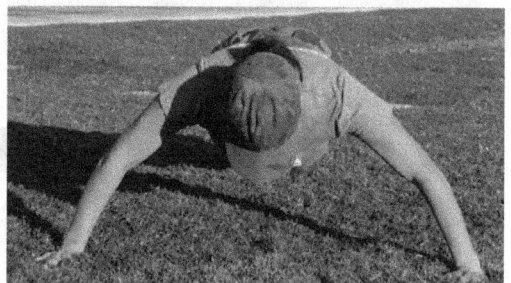

Sarge – Show the group how to do wide pushups!
Bend those elbows keep your head up!

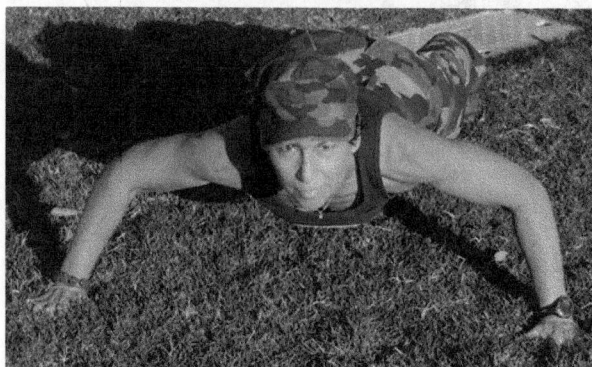

8-Count Body Builder Pushups

Position 1

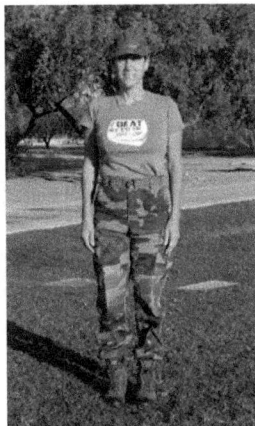

Position 2

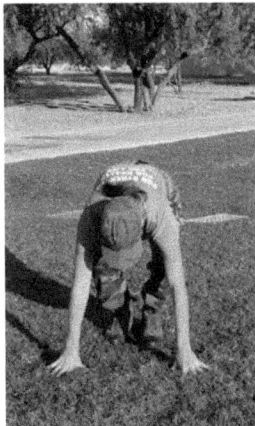

Position 3

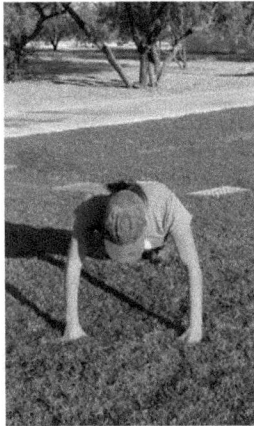

Position 4

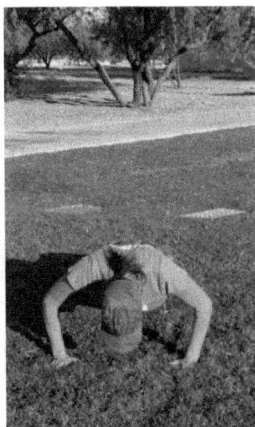

Position5

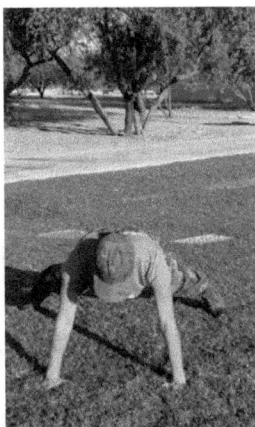

Position 6

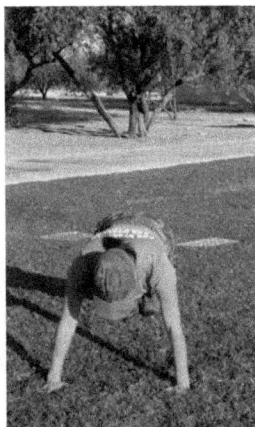

Position 7

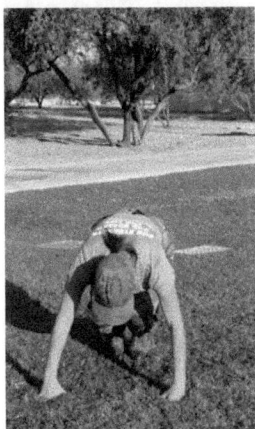

Position 8

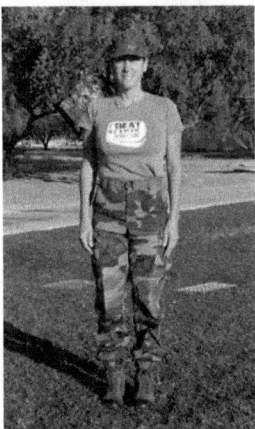

Name: Margo Susco
Age: 45
Buddy
# of Years in BCBC: 1 year
Occupation: Small Business Owner
Something of Interest: Love Classic
Cars, Drag Racing, Motorcycles,
Big Band Music, and Ballroom
Dancing

Pushup Rows — Lie on the ground with dumbbells in your hand placed next to your chest. Your hands should be shoulder width apart. Push yourself up by doing a pushup. Lift your left arm up next to your chest like you were doing a row. Bring it back down and repeat with the other arm. Do a pushup again and repeat.

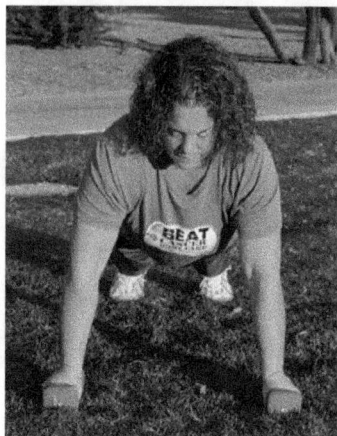

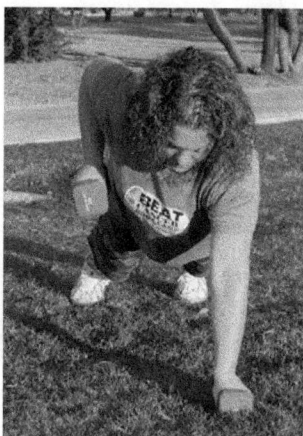

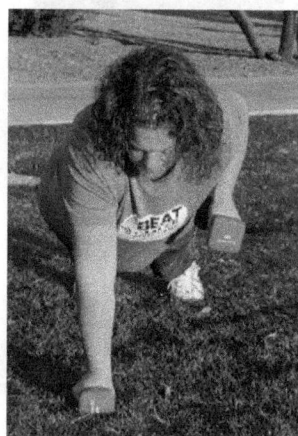

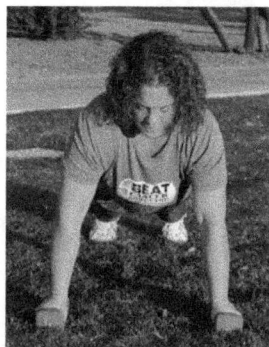

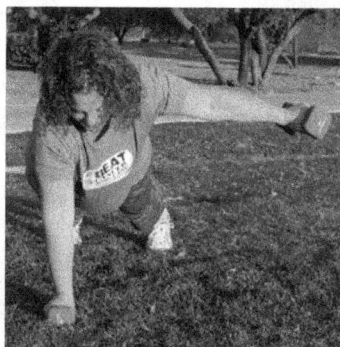

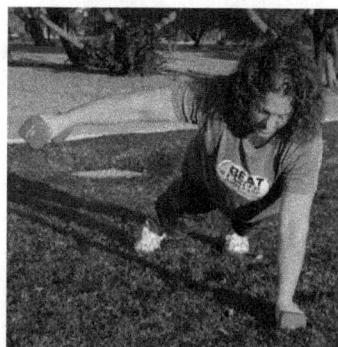

Pushup Flies — Lie on the ground with dumbbells in your hand placed next to your chest. Your hands should be shoulder width apart. Push yourself up by doing a pushup. Lift your left arm up and extend it out to the side. Bring it back down and repeat with the other arm. Do a pushup again and repeat.

Name: Tami Ballis
Age: 43
Buddy
How long in BCBC: 6 months
Occupation: Branch Manager, Professional Staffing Services
Something of Interest: I enjoy spending quality time with friends and family. I am passionate about quality of life ... making every day count and living life to the fullest!

Day 1 Crunch Cycle –10 each *Walk/run /bike – 15:00 Full body stretch	**Day 2** Repeat 5 times Pushups –10/ Crunches –10 Shoulder workout Walk 15:00 Full body stretch	**Day 3** Repeat 5 times Walk / run or bike – 3:00 squats - 20 Full body stretch	**Day 4** Repeat 5 times Bicep curls/ triceps ext – 10 Shoulder workout Walk / run / bike – 15:00 Full body stretch	**Day 5** Crunch Cycle – 10 each Walk / run / bike – 15:00 Full body stretch
Day 6 Repeat 5 times Walk / run or bike - 3:00 squats – 20 lunges –10 Full body stretch	**Day 7** Crunch Cycle – 15 each Walk / run or bike – 15:00 Full body stretch	**Day 8** Repeat 5 times Jumping jacks 10 Pushups – 5-10 Shoulder Workout Full body stretch	**Day 9** Repeat 3 times Walk or bike 5:00 squats – 20 lunge-10/leg Full body stretch	**Day 10** Crunch Cycle 15 each Shoulder workout walk / run / bike – 15:00 Full body stretch
Day 11 Plank pose 1:00 Walk / run / bike – 15:00 – Do 20 squats every 3 minutes Full body stretch	**Day 12** Repeat 5 times Jumping jacks 10 Pushups – 5-10 Shoulder workout Full body stretch	**Day 13** Crunch Cycle – 15 each Walk / run / bike – 15:00 – do 20 squats every 3 minutes Full body stretch	**Day 14** Repeat 5 times jumping jacks – 10 Pushups – 10 Shoulder Workout Full body stretch	**Day 15** Crunch Cycle – 15 reps Walk / run / bike – 15:00 Full body stretch
Day 16 Repeat 5 times Bicep curls/tricep ext – 10 squats – 20 lunges – 10 Shoulder Workout Full body stretch	**Day 17** Crunch Cycle – 15 reps Walk/run/bike – 15:00 Full body stretch	**Day 18** Repeat 5 times Pushups – 10 Squats – 20 Shoulder Workout Full body stretch	**Day 19** Crunch Cycle – 15 reps walk/run/bike – 15:00 Full body stretch	**Day 20** Repeat 5 times Pushups – 10 Squats – 10-20 crunches – 20 Full body stretch
Day 21 Shoulder Workout Crunch cycle – 15 reps Walk/run/bike – 15:00 Full body stretch	**Day 22** Repeat 8 times jumping jacks – 10 pushups – 5-10 Bench dips 10-15 Full body stretch	**Day 23** Crunch Cycle – 15 reps Walk/run/bike – 15:00 Full body stretch	**Day 24** Repeat 5 times Pushups - 10-15 Squats - 20/ Crunches– 20 Shoulder Workout Full body stretch	**Day 25** Crunch Cycle – 20 reps walk / run / bike - 15:00 Full body stretch

Explanation of the workout charts

The Twenty Five Day Beginner Plan — This is a great guide to start moving again — complete with stretching, walking, and light weights and calisthenics to prepare for the more rigorous routine that follows. The goal of the 25 day plan is to build a habit of fitting fitness back into your life. You can choose to do the 25 days straight through or opt to do five days a week for five weeks.

In the 25 day workout below, you will see "Repeat 5–10 times" many times in the workout of the day. Basically, repeat the events under the above phrase until you reach another line or space in between the exercises of the workout for that day. Exercises like Bike 10–20:00 or Crunch Cycle, full body stretch, or shoulder workout ARE NOT to be repeated several times — JUST DO THEM ONCE.

Walk/run/bike — 15:00 — This is your cardio exercise choice. Some people prefer to swim, row, bike over walking or running. It is up to you. Get moving and do something for that day. If you wish you can even pick more than one option to do for that day and mix in a walk with a bike or a swim even.

Plank — 1:00 — you will see 1 minute next to the plank pose — try to see how long you can hold the plank and build up to 1 minute.

***The 25 Day Chart is the daily minimal amount of recommended exercise you need to do in this workout plan. ***

The Five Week Plan — The next pages after the chart is the more intermediate/ advanced program and has additional exercise to assist with fat burning and abdominal toning. It is designed to give you two workouts per week of calisthenics and light weight routines plus one or more cardio only workouts. The cardio options are your choice — walk, run, swim, bike, play a sport like tennis, or anything that will allow for you to burn extra calories.

Week 1

Workout #1
Upper body Workout

Walk or jog 5:00
Stretch
(LWS) Light Weight Shoulders — 3-5lbs
Repeat 3 times
Bicep curls — 10-15 reps
Tricep ext — 10-15 reps
Military press — 10-15 reps
Assisted pull-ups — max reps
*Pushups — 5 - 10
Crunches — 20
Chest press — 10-15 reps
Arm Haulers — 20
Birds — 20
Reverse pushups —20
*any variety = knee, wide,
regular, tricep etc.
Cardio option of choice — 20-30 min
Stretch

Workout #2
Full body Workout

Walk, jog, or bike 10:00
Leg exercises:
Repeat 2-3 times
Squats — 10-20
½ squats — 10-20
Lunges — 10/leg
Heel raises — 20/leg
Dirty dogs — 20/leg
Bike or Cardio 5:00
Hammer curls — 10-15 reps
Tricep ext — 10-15 reps
Reverse flies — 10-15
Military press — 10-15 reps
*if you wish you can replace leg
calisthenics with machine weights:
Leg extensions,
Leg curls, and
Leg press,
Cardio option of walking, biking,
elliptical glide, swimming 15-20 min

Supplemental Training (do 2-3 times per week)
Stretch Program - 10 minutes
Walk or cardio of choice - 20-30 min
Repeat one of the workouts on this page for a 3rd workout/week

Week 2

Workout #1
Full body
Walk 5:00/stretch
Repeat Circuit 3 times
Hammer curls — 10-15 reps
Tricep ext — 10-15 reps
Reverse flies — 10-15
Military press — 10-15 reps
Assisted Pullups — max reps
Rest with crunches — 25 reps
Pushups — 10-20 (on knees if necessary/variety)
Bench Dips — 10-15
Squats — 20
Lunges — 10/leg
Heel raises — 20
Dirty dogs — 20/leg
Walk, jog, bike 5:00
Cardio option 20-30 minutes
Light weight shoulders:
Lateral raise — 10
  thumbs up — 10
  thumbs down — 10
Front raise — 10
Cross overheads — 10 (like jumping jack motion)
Overhead press — 10

Workout #2
Upper body
Warmup bike/walk — total 10:00
Stretch
Repeat 3 times
Cardio — 5 minutes, but make each minute harder than the previous (increase speed, resistance, incline etc)
Hammer curls — 10-15 reps
Tricep ext — 10-15 reps
Reverse flies — 10-15
Military press — 10-15 reps
Reverse Flies — 10
Birds — 20
Reverse pushups — 20
Arm Haulers — 20
Chest press — 15 reps (w/DB)
Bent over Rows — 15 reps (w/DB)
Light weight Shoulder — 10 reps each 3-5# DBs
Walk or cardio of choice — 10 minute cooldown and Stretch

Supplemental Training (do 2-3 times per week)
Stretch Program - 10 minutes
Walk or cardio of choice - 20-30 min
Repeat one of the workouts on this page for a 3rd workout/week

---

Week 3

Workout #1

Walk or jog 5:00
Repeat 5 times
Jumping Jacks — 10
Squats — 10
Pushups — 5-10
Stretch
Lightweight Shoulders — 5 lbs
Repeat 3 times
Walk 5 minutes
Hammer curls — 10-15 reps
Tricep ext — 10-15 reps
Reverse flies — 10-15
Squats — 20
Heel raises — 20
Bench Dips — 10-15
Chest press —15-20 reps (w/DB)
Reverse Pushups — 20
Birds — 20
Pushups — 10-15
Assisted Pullups max reps
Rows — 15 reps (w/DB)
Lightweight Shoulder 3-5 lbs
Crunch cycle — 20/set
Cardio option of choice 20-30 minutes

Workout #2

Warmup 5 minutes walk
Stretch
Repeat 3 times
Hammer curls — 10-15 reps
Tricep ext — 10-15 reps
Reverse flies — 10-15
Military press — 10-15 reps
Chest Press — 15 reps with DB
Rows — 15 reps with DB
Squats — 20
Lunges 10/leg
Heel raises — 20
Dirty dogs — 25/leg
Upperbody Cycle (1 time thru)
Chest press — 15
Assisted Pullups — 10
Bent Over Rows — 15
Bicep curls — 15
Military press — 15
Pushup / Rows — 5/arm w/DB
Bench Dips — 10-15
Walk 10 minutes
Stretch

Supplemental Training (do 2-3 times per week)
Stretch Program - 10 minutes
Walk or cardio of choice - 20-30 min
Repeat one of the workouts on this page for a 3rd workout/week

Week 4

Workout #1

Repeat 5 times
Jumping Jacks — 10
Squats — 15
Pushups — 5-10
Repeat 4-5 times
Walk, jog or bike 3 minutes
Squats — 20
Lunges — 20/leg
Heel Raises — 20
Dirty Dogs — 20/leg
Bear crawls — 20 yds
Repeat 4 times
Walk, jog or bike 3 minutes
Bench dips — 20
Abs of choice — 20
Pushups — 10-20 or
Chest Press — 10-20
Assisted pull-ups — max reps
Lightweight Shoulders 5 lbs
Cooldown stretch
Crunch Cycle (advanced)
Crunches — 25
Reverse Crunches — 25
Double Crunches — 25
Left Crunches — 25
Right Crunches — 25
Bicycle Crunches — 25
Flutterkicks — 20
Leg Levers — 20
Hip rolls — 20 (10 each side)
Plank Pose 1 min

Workout #2

Crunch cycle — 20/exercise
Regular Crunch — shoulders blades off floor
Reverse Crunch — hips off floor
Double Crunch — both hips / shoulders off floor at the same time
Left crunches — 20
Right crunches — 20 (elbow toward opposite knees)
Plank pose 30 seconds
Stretch stomach
Lightweight Shoulders
Dumbbells/PT: Repeat 3 times
Chest Press — 15
Bent Over Row — 15
Bench Dips — 15
Assisted pull-ups — max reps
Cooldown w/Abs
Walk — 15-20 minutes

Supplemental Training (do 2-3 times per week)
Stretch Program - 10 minutes
Walk or cardio of choice - 20-30 min
Repeat one of the workouts on this page for a 3rd workout/week

Week 5

Workout #1

Crunch Cycle — 25 per set
Repeat 5 times
Jumping Jacks — 10
Squats — 20
Stretch 30 seconds
Lightweight Shoulder
Squats — 15
Pushups — 15
Lunges — 10/leg
Bicep curls — 15
Heel raises — 25
Bent Over rows — 15
Assisted Pullups - 10
Walk, Jog, Bike 5 minutes
Mixed Circuit
Half Squats — 20
Chest Press — 20
Half Lunges — 15/leg
Bent Over Rows — 15
Heel raises — 25
Dirty Dogs — 20/leg
Bear Crawls 20 yds
Walk, Jog, Bike 5 minutesPlank
Pose — 1 min
Pushups — max reps
Hammer curls — 10-15 reps
Tricep ext — 10-15 reps
Reverse flies — 10-15
Military press — 10-15 reps
Chest Press — 15 reps
Bent Over Rows — 15
Cooldown 10 minutes walk
Stretch

Workout #2

Walk 5 minutes
Repeat 5 times
Jumping Jacks — 10
Squats — 20
Pushups — 5-10
Mixed Circuit
Bicep Curls — 15
Squats — 25
Tricep Ext — 15
Lunges — 15/leg
Chest press — 15
Plank Pose 1 min
Assisted Pullups — 15
Bent Over Rows — 15
Dumbbell Circuit
Chest Press — 15
Bent Over Rows — 15/arm
Pushup — flies — 5/arm
Pushups — rows — 5/arm
Lightweight Shoulders — 5 lbs
Repeat Mixed Circuit above
Crunches Cycle — 20 reps each

Supplemental Training (do 2-3 times per week)
Stretch Program - 10 minutes
Walk or cardio of choice - 20-30 min
Repeat one of the workouts on this page for a 3rd workout/week

Chapter Eight: Commit To Be Fit

Some time ago, I was approached by a local news anchor, Martha Vasquez, to be a regular on her newscast. She was familiar with my program, and even attended some classes. Her good friend is a member o the group, and she hears all about it. I mentioned to her how I would love to be able to reach out to more people in a non-threatening, friendly way. I wanted to show them exercise doesn't have to be rocket science, or take up a big chunk of your day.

At first, my appearance on her show was to be taped once a week. We'd film a little snippet of an exercise that I could demonstrate how to do anywhere, anytime. We decided this segment should be called "Commit to be Fit."

This show aired weekly on Fridays. Almost a year into it, we discussed a better way to reach out to the audience. A one-minute segment was nice and informative, but appearing on-air live to discuss the exercise was even better. We then changed it to every other week, but I would be on set to discuss the exercise I demonstrated.

At first, I feared it would be nerve-wracking to be on live TV, but Martha is such a professional that she made me feel like I was talking with a friend, not on a set surrounded by cameras. I now film the segments in various locations, and then go to the studio the Fridays it airs. It is a great way to help educate and promote everyday exercises that can be done anywhere.

We'd tape the segment in a grocery store one day, the next day in a gas station. Come on, we all know that everyone has to shop some time or another, so make the most of it. How about pumping gas? Why just stand there and watch the numbers go up on the tank? Do something that would feel good — exercise while you're waiting! I get a kick out of it when people tell me that they actually do some of these exercises. It would be great one day to see more people not being embarrassed but instead proud of exercising, and doing it anywhere, anytime!

One of the most common concerns I hear is that there is just no time to exercise. Believe me, I wish the days were a little longer, so I could get more things done, too. Realistically, that won't happen, so it's best to find time to exercise while you are already doing something. That's called multi tasking. It is really not that hard to do. I will show you a few ways to sneak that exercise you've been longing to do into your schedule. Hell, you might end up even exercising more than you thought you could ever do.

Another key component to exercise is to find ways to always shake it up a bit. This way you won't get bored. Yea, I know most of these are basic exercises, but they are the ones that really work best. They are tried and true over the decades. The key is finding different variations and locations that they could be done. That will make it successful when you incorporate it into your everyday schedule. There is no excuse not to do these, when you already have the time … you just didn't know it. Finding various locations is keeps things fresh. Looking around your surroundings it is fun to imagine everything as potential exercise equipment. Who needs a gym? Who needs machines? We are machines!

Commit To be Fit – Exercises
Let's just start with some basic advice to get it out of the way. WALK. Unless you live in some remote area and you don't feel it's safe, always park your car far away and walk. It amazes me how much time people waste driving around the parking lots, circling the aisles in hope of finding that perfect spot two feet from the door. Not only did they waste at least ten minutes of their time, they are probably all stressed out from that, and not feeling very happy by now. On the other hand, there are usually spaces far away where you could pull right in and happily walk into the store. Stress free! Keep your abs tight, swing your arms, and you're already starting your workout!

Here are other ideas and ways to work exercise into your everyday lifestyle.

Knee ups — while standing by refrigerator, before you open the fridge to look for some snacks … think twice. Do some knee ups. Hold on to the refrigerator door for balance. Try doing 10 on each side. Stop rethink what you were going to take out and eat. Now repeat the sequence. Bet you won't be so hungry.

Squats — do while brushing your teeth. What a perfect time to get some squats in. You probably brush your teeth at least twice a day. Do 20 squats each time. If you are uncoordinated, please take the toothbrush out of your mouth while squatting!

Lunges — stationary, foot up on parking curb. A parking lot, is a great place to put your leg up, and do some stationary lunges. Using a parking block, or step, do 20 lunges each side.

Calf Raises — while on the phone. I know how much time is spent on the phone, while make the most of it. Do calf raises while talking. If you are on hold, even better try doing them double time!

Triceps Dips — park bench, chairs, boulders, Just about any place you could get your hands on you can do tricep dips. The intensity will vary depending on the height of the item. Don't worry, just remember, good form, elbows go back.

Seated Abs — do on park benches or chairs. You don't need to lay down on the floor to do crunches or work out your abs. You can get a good workout by sitting. On a chair or bench, keep your feet on the ground, and slowly lean back until you feel your abs contract. Now hold that position, and then sit up. Do that 15 times, and you will begin to feel it work. If it's nice out, go for a walk in the park, and do some this on a park bench.

Bicep curls — with watering cans. Watering your plants you could do some bicep curls first. With the cans pretty full, they will act as some weights, and help you gain strength in your biceps.

Triceps kickbacks — do with water bottles. It is always good to work the opposing muscles, so sneak in some tricep kickbacks. Make sure there is some weight to the water bottles.

Lateral raises — do with books, copy paper. This is one that is easy to do with many things. You want to be able to grasp an item in your hands, so you don't drop your items. Heavy books, and copy paper usually work well for these, and you can almost always find some at work.

Step ups — park bench, curbs. What a great way to get some cardio in and some fresh air at the same time. If you find it pretty easy doing these on a curb, challenge yourself and do some on a bench. Watch your footing. You can do it!

Pushwups — walls, tables, stairs. Ahh.push-ups. My favorite. These can be done anywhere! There is always a wall, a bench, table, or even stairs, to do some modified push-ups. As you gain strength, you will eventually be able to do some on the ground, and finally do the full military style.

Pull ups — low bars. At a park, perhaps, you will find dip bars, which a perfect alternative to start doing pull-ups. You can keep your feet on the ground, bend your knees, and use your body weight to pull up.

Commit To be Fit - A Typical day of exercise
As I mentioned, the key to sneaking fitness in your routine is to be creative! Don't let surroundings dictate what you can do! Let me share with you some ways to get your daily fitness in whether you are at work, shopping, or even at the gas station. Here is

a typical day, that even without going to a gym, you could have a great workout.

So let's say you are on your way to work, and realize you need to stop for gas in your car. I say perfect! While you are filling up your car..get busy! Begin by doing calf raises on the curb. Try doing 20 or so. Next, move to the bumper of your car, and get ready to do some tricep dips. Do 10. stretch. Repeat. If you have a big gas guzzler, and you're still waiting, do some cardio step ups on the curb. Hurry up … don't be late for work.

When you get to work, now the fun begins. Don't even think of taking an elevator. Start climbing the stairs, and MOVE IT! You say your office is on the first floor, well run up the stairs and say "good morning" to someone above you! Now get to your desk! Before you start your work day, do 15 modified push-ups on your desk. Stretch your arms. 10 more can't hurt. If I were you, I'd do some work now …

Time to go to the copy room. Lucky you. Pick up a package of paper, and before you fill up the copy machine, let's use it as weights. That's right, using one side first, do 10 single arm rows, followed by lateral raises. Now switch sides. Look around … what can you use for tricep extensions? Hmmm, how about a stapler, or 3 ring hole punch? Anything with a little weight will do the trick, after all you're just going to sneak in perhaps 15-20 extensions. By this time you're thinking of your lunch break. Good thing you brought some leftovers to work to heat up in the microwave. Guess what? Now you will challenge yourself by doing wall squats while waiting for your food to heat up. With your back against the wall, hold the squat position while you wait. I bet you're happy, you don't have a big meal to heat up! Don't just stand there, alternate raising your heels. Whew. That was good!

Remember to keep hydrating, and bring some bottles of water back to your desk. It is so important to drink water, and to always have a few bottles with you. Not only is it good for you, but they could double as weights. Time to do some bicep curls with them. Alternating arms, nice and slow do 20 curls. Now do 10 curls together. The next exercise will be tricep kick backs. Keep using the bottles as weights, and do 15 on each side. If you still have some time, repeat the sequence. Time to get back to work.

Don't be upset you have to stop at the grocery store on the way home, it is a great place to work on your lunges. What a perfect place to stroll down the aisles with your cart, and nice and slow, do some walking lunges. Having the cart to help you balance you could concentrate on some good form. If you are using a small hand held basket, instead, great. As you fill it up with groceries, do some hammer curls. If the basket is not too heavy, alternate some front raises.

Hurry home, it's dinner time! Before you eat, do some tricep dips on your chair. Be very careful that the chair is sturdy,and most importantly, doesn't have wheels! After you are done with dinner, and you are cleaning up, take out a broom and sweep your floor. Don't stop there. Use your broom to do some military presses. You could easily do 20 of these in no time. Ahhh — time for a break. Catch the news on TV. On the commercial break, do crunches for your abs, and then alternate some push-ups. Do 10 of each until the news comes back on. It's almost time to end the day, so as you prepare for bed, sneak in some good stretches.

Not bad, for not going to the gym! Good job. There is always tomorrow to challenge yourself in more creative ways to exercise.

"The question isn't who is going to let me; it's who's going to stop me."

- Ayn Rand

Chapter Nine: Strength in Numbers

Take Charge

There is strength in numbers. Imagine you are training to run a marathon. It is difficult to train by yourself, because you're not accountable to teammates who depend upon you to show up and work. Once you make the commitment to meet others, you feel the responsibility to stay disciplined and focus on your goals.

The big day of the marathon finally arrives, and you are out there with thousands of other runners. You are half way through the race, and feel like giving up. Along comes a runner keeping pace with you. This is a total stranger. You immediately connect with her and continue to run together, cheering each other on. Pushing each other to keep going. You might have even given up, and walked, but you didn't want to disappoint her, or is it the little competitive spark that pushes you? How strange, you barely know her, maybe know her first name. You keep running along side of each other, talking up a storm and learning all about her. Hell, you have 13 miles to go.

Along comes another group of runners, and now you're all talking, laughing, sharing stories. Funny, it first started that the only common bond was that you were all running the same race. That was enough to feel connected while you continue to encourage each other to keep going — not stopping until you reach that finish line!

Fighting cancer is like running a marathon. You have to remain strong, push yourself to cross that finish line, and don't be afraid to get the support and encouragement of others. Most people don't enjoy being alone, especially when the unknown can be so scary. Unfortunately that sometimes happens with family and friends. They mean well, but don't know how to handle the situation. Sometimes they might even avoid talking about the diagnosis, or even withdraw completely, leaving you feeling all alone. This is when it is so important to find people you can talk to, and connect with what you are going through. This is not the time to feel you have to be brave or tough it out on your own. This is when you need the support of people to help you move forward. Keep running. One foot in front of the other, and don't stop until you cross the finish line.

There is something almost magical when you put a diverse group of people together for a common cause ... beat cancer! Not only do strength, laughter, and knowledge multiply, but so does the energy! The dynamics in the group constantly change. There is virtually nothing that we can't accomplish as a group. We are not afraid to lean on each other when needed, and pull others up when they're feeling down. Everything is shared with each other. Secrets are kept within our group. The bond is like super glue.

How fortunate to have such a large pool of women together to share their stories. Nothing is off limits. They talk about the doctors they have consulted, and those that they choose not to use. It is very informative to hear firsthand the truth. Sometimes it's not always pleasant. So many questions, so many things to learn. In the past the only choices they had was to look at pictures from the doctor's office to see what reconstruction looks like. Let's be honest, do you really think any doctor is going to photograph a patient with poor results? Or even talk about the horror stories? That would be professional suicide. Well ... along comes Boot Camp, we have nothing to hide. On the contrary, we want to help others make smart, educated decisions.

And there are no holds barred.

One day when we were having our monthly lunch in a private room at a restaurant. The topic of conversation for the day was breast reconstruction. There were many people there who had it done, and a few more contemplating the procedure. What could have been a better setting to share this wealth of information than at the restaurant, over lunch. I felt it was almost the fashion show of breasts.

One by one, members lined up to lift up their shirts to show off their latest addition. They walked their own catwalk, stopping, posing, then whirling around. It was quite a sight, especially when the young waiter caught a glimpse of it all. He really didn't know what to make of it all even though he knew we were a cancer support group. He quickly closed the doors to the private room, and handed me some napkins to hold up over the glass doors for more privacy. I'm sure we quickly got the reputation of being a wild group.

While we were having coffee after one of our get-togethers, the hot topic of reconstruction came up once again. A proud member graciously offered to show her reconstructed breasts. The best way to learn what they looks like is to see them in person, not pictures. So we get up close and personal! We all anxiously wait for her to lift up her shirt. She then unhooks her bra, to expose her breasts. We all ooh and ahh at how nice they really look. It sure puts these women at ease to know how breasts can look after this type of surgery.

One of the members is so intrigued, she asks, "May I touch it?"

After all how does anyone know what a reconstructed breast feels like? This is important. Of course the lady says, sure. She is a bit apprehensive about all this. I believe this was the first time someone other than her doctor, or husband were so interested. But in the Boot Camp spirit, and really wanting to help out she agrees.

After some touching and squeezing the interested member was relieved and said, "Wow, it feels real good." The troop member quietly answers, "Thanks, but that was my real breast!" We all burst out laughing. Go figure, she never mentioned she only had one breast reconstructed!

The "Healing Circle" was introduced to me when I was on a retreat that several of us from Beat Cancer Boot Camp attended. I had walked by myself one evening to a Native American ceremony being held under the stars. I sat among other survivors and oncology nurses that were attending the retreat who I had not yet met. The experience was overwhelming.

We sat as strangers but that circle created the most amazing bond. When we all joined hands and thought quietly to ourselves about the energy from the circle and it's healing powers, I was moved beyond words. When it was over, the first thing I thought of was that I wanted to share this with my fellow Boot Campers. If there was this kind of positive energy when you did this with strangers I could only imagine what it would be with my very dear friends.

This past May, our Beat Cancer Boot Camp went on our yearly retreat. We spent three wonderful days together. At the conclusion of our weekend our group went on a "Pink Jeep Tour" of the beautiful Sedona, AZ area. Towards the end of the tour we found ourselves overlooking a spectacular vista point and we decided to do the "Healing circle" as our final bonding moment.

There were about 35 of us that formed a huge circle. We even included the jeep drivers. We all closed our eyes and I just told everyone to just think good thoughts. "Pray if you pray, send good vibes around the circle or just think about the power of healing as a group".

We had a moment of complete silence (if you knew this group you would know how difficult that is). I knew that this was such a very special moment in my life but honestly, I just didn't know what the reaction of the rest of the group would be. We opened our eyes, looked around the circle and all of a sudden I would say that 80% of us were weeping. Everyone started hugging and said how amazing it had felt to be a part of something so special.

- Pam J.

All of that exercise, friendship, and support is not worth much if you're eating hot dogs and potato chips for lunch every day. Let's see what we eat in the Beat Cancer Beat Camp mess hall!

Chapter Ten: Beat Cancer Boot Camp Mess Hall

Take Charge of your Diet

OK, we occasionally serve pizza and bagels at some of our meals, but we've been exercising. If we had a full-time mess hall, this is how we would feed you. Our plan is to help you maintain your energy, build muscles, stay hydrated, stay healthy, and stay at a healthy weight. We would help you understand that nourishing yourself, even after a diagnosis of cancer, can be easy.

The Big Picture

The world of nutrition advice has its share of confusion and contradiction. And when you're dealing with your health, you don't want to get it wrong. That's why we consulted the experts. They want you to know that even though there are some unanswered questions, the big picture of healthy eating is pretty clear. And it doesn't mean you have to give up any of the pleasure of eating.

The big picture isn't just about what you eat. It is also about how you think about eating and food. Consider these thoughts.

Nourishing yourself is like exercise in several ways. First, they both keep you healthy. Second, the both require commitment and self-discipline. Supermarkets today sell both the healthiest and the unhealthiest foods you can find. If you try to navigate this confusing world of food without following some rules, you're likely to be in trouble. It pays to have some "I never eat" and "I always eat" rules to guide you.

Everyone is different. Not only do we have different styles of eating and favorite flavors and textures, but we also have unique nutritional needs. The broad advice we offer here about what and how to eat applies to everyone. Because of our differences, it is perfectly acceptable for your rules about eating to be different than someone else's.

One overall rule we offer up that can apply to everyone is to eat real food. We like the advice of avoiding foods your grandmother wouldn't recognize, foods with ingredients you can't pronounce.

With that out of the way, let's move on to some specifics.

Eat for Energy and Exercise Food is fuel for your body, the fuel you burn when you exercise. It also provides the raw materials for building new muscle, healing injuries and replacing the cells in your body that have had their run. It even has a direct effect on blood sugar, insulin and the neurotransmitters that influence how you feel. Following some simple guidelines can keep an inconsistent eating pattern from compromising your energy. It can help you build a stronger body and have more stamina.

Eat breakfast every day. You may not need a lot of food in the morning. You may not need to eat right when you get up. You don't need to eat traditional breakfast food. But nourishing yourself within a couple of hours of rising will jump start your metabolism and give you some fuel to run on. Experiment with what makes you feel best, but avoid sugary pastries or cereals.

Eat on a regular schedule. We often recommend eating every 4 hours during the day, but you can discover a schedule that works best for you. Don't go for long periods of time without eating. It always catches up with you, either resulting in low energy or overeating later in the day.

Slow-carb foods:
Oats Whole wheat pasta Beans Apples and pears Sweet potato

Eat before and after your Boot Camp workout. About an hour to 45 minutes before you exercise, have a small snack that provides some slow-carb and protein. Slow-carbs have a low glycemic index. They are digested slowly and give you a source of sustained fuel while you exercise. The protein begins the process of digestion and will be available in your body after exercise to help build and repair muscle.

After exercise, within twenty minutes or so, have another snack providing some fast-carb and protein. Fast-carbs have a high glycemic index. They are digested quickly and can start replacing glycogen in your muscles. Glycogen is a form of carbohydrate in your muscles and liver that your body uses for quick energy during exercise. The protein is again used to build and repair muscle.

Fast-carb foods:
Orange juice or other Baked potato Rice Banana Melon Mango

Good pre-exercise snacks:
After exercise, within twenty minutes or so, have another snack providing some fast-carb and protein. Fast-carbs have a high glycemic index. They are digested quickly and can start replacing glycogen in your muscles. Glycogen is a form of carbohydrate in your muscles and liver that your body uses for quick energy during exercise. The protein is again used to build and repair muscle.

Water is extremely important for the functioning of every cell and system in the body. The old rule of drinking 8 glasses of water a day doesn't hold true for everyone, but some guidelines are helpful in staying hydrated. As with other aspects of your nutrition, your fluid needs are quite individual. When we are not exercising or out in summer heat, most of us get enough. But when we start a program like Boot Camp, we should start paying more attention.

Get in the habit of drinking water throughout the day. Establish a routine like reaching for water at ten in the morning and two in the afternoon, in addition to your other drinking occasions.

Eat lots of vegetables and fruits every day. These foods are filled with water and provide almost half of the fluid our bodies use most days.

Look at the color. A good gauge of hydration on days you don't exercise is to drink enough to maintain light yellow urine. Remember though, even if you are well hydrated, if you take a multi or B vitamins your urine will be dark yellow.

Weigh yourself. The best way to tell how much fluid you need when you exercise is to weigh yourself before and after a typical workout. The weight loss you see is from fluid loss. It needs to be replaced by drinking before, during and after exercise. Keep your water bottle with you and remember that one cup of water or 8 fluid ounces weighs about one half pound.

Skip the sweet ones. You can count beverages other than water, although we recommend limiting sweetened beverages because of the sugar and calories. Beverages sweetened with artificial sweeteners are tempting, but you are probably better off with water or plain tea for most of your fluid intake.

Be a sport? Sports beverages generally contain sugar and electrolytes, both of which help the absorption of water from the drink. They are okay to drink during exercise, but diluted fruit juice has the same effect. They are too caloric to drink when you're not exercising.

These can add subtle flavor to a bottle of plain water:

Orange, lemon, or lime
Cucumber
Fresh ginger
Fresh mint
Fresh basil

What about green tea?

There are lots of scientific reasons to think that green tea can help fight cancer and other diseases. It is especially rich in catechins, compounds that have many disease fighting properties. Unfortunately, definitive research studies showing green tea's protection against cancer just haven't been done. Nonetheless, green tea is a wise beverage of choice, if you like it. Brew it yourself, though, because bottled teas have far less of the beneficial catechins and can be loaded with sugar or artificial sweeteners.

And - what about alcohol?

Alcoholic beverages are never recommended as a means to stay hydrated for obvious reasons. But many people who have had cancer, especially women with breast cancer, wonder if an occasional drink is okay. The answer to this just isn't clear, and it feels like a lot is at stake.

Research certainly shows that even moderate alcohol intake (like a drink a day) is associated with a real increased risk of breast cancer, as well as other cancers. The effect of drinking alcohol after a diagnosis still isn't clear. We think it is a good idea to be cautious. We are anxious to see what future research shows.

Eat to stay healthy

A high quality diet is essential to staying healthy after a cancer diagnosis. Although there are lots of questions about the effect of certain foods on cancer, researchers are finding that a pattern of eating is more than the sum of its parts. Your pattern may have more impact than the presence or absence of individual foods. Two healthy patterns of eating are the Prudent diet and the Mediterranean diet. As a comparison, the Western diet is in all cases linked to more disease.

The Prudent diet pattern focuses on these foods:	
Vegetables of all kinds	Tomatoes
Fruits and fruit juices	Legumes (beans)
Fish	Soups
Whole grains	Poultry (not fried)
Rice, grains and pasta	Nuts
Cold cereals	

The Mediterranean diet pattern focuses on these foods:	
Vegetables	Fruits
Fish	Whole grains
Olive oil	Nuts
Yogurt or cheese	Little red meat

The Western diet pattern focuses on these foods:	
Red meat	Processed meat
Creamy soups and sauces	Butter
Mayonnaise	Fried potatoes
Fried chicken	High fat dairy foods
Snacks	Refined grains
Pasta or potato salads	High-calorie drinks / sweets

Look closely at the descriptions of these three patterns and you'll see why the Prudent and Mediterranean patterns trump the Western one. Studies show that people whose eating patterns more closely fit the healthy patterns are healthier themselves. But does that mean that a healthy eater never eats a hamburger? For some, it does mean that. For others, an occasional hamburger doesn't completely disrupt their intention to eat well.

We all make dozens of food choices each week. What matters most is your choice the majority of the time you're shopping or perusing a menu. More healthy food choices are better. Less unhealthy food choices are better. But you knew that. What is difficult is keeping track of the times we give ourselves permission to indulge in something unhealthy.

We encourage you to practice mindful eating. Each time you make a food choice, make sure you are making a conscious decision. Consider the consequences. Consider how your choices fit with your intentions.

The parts of the healthy patterns: Vegetables and fruit
Vegetables and fruit may well be the most important aspect of a healthy diet when it comes to beating cancer and otherwise staying healthy. It is safe to say that it should be a priority.

How much do you need each day?

Most studies show that more is always better than less. In other words, the people that eat the most have a dramatic advantage over those that eat the least. The people at the high end in the studies are generally consuming a total of 8 to 10 servings of produce each day. But there is also no doubt that meeting the 5-a-day rule provides more protection than eating fewer servings.

What is a serving?

Although there is no hard and fast rule, the simplest approach favored by most nutritionists is to consider a serving as ½ cup of vegetables and fruit, with the exception of salad greens, for which the serving size is 2 cups. The relatively modest size of ½ cup makes it easier to accumulate 8 to 10 servings a day. One helpful strategy is to dish up a larger portion of cooked vegetable, like a full cup of broccoli.

Which vegetables and fruits are best?

Different vegetables and fruit have unique protective qualities so choosing a wide variety is our advice. The pigments that give produce its array of colors are beneficial, hence the recommendation to eat for color. Remember, though, that onion, garlic and cauliflower — three decidedly white vegetables — are potent disease fighters.

At the top of the lists:

Vegetables	Fruit
Leafy greens, both cooked and raw	Berries of all kinds
Cruciferous vegetables like broccoli, cauliflower, cabbage	Citrus
	Apples and pears
Tomatoes (okay, technically a fruit)	Bananas
Carrots	Peaches, plums, apricots
Onion, garlic and leeks	
Mushrooms	

What about organic?

This is a good question. First of all, it is important to understand that eating generous amounts of vegetables and fruit is a higher priority than eating only organic, in our minds. Virtually all the large observational studies that relate how people eat to their risk of most cancers show that those who eat more vegetables and fruit have a significantly lower risk than those who eat less. Most of those studies were done in a time when organic produce was not as available as it is today. The conclusion we draw is that even conventionally grown product is protective.

On the other hand, both experts and consumers are concerned about exposure to pesticide residues and believe that we should avoid them when we can.

Often, eating exclusively organic is not an option. Both cost and availability are limiting factors. In that case, knowing which vegetables and fruit have the most pesticide residues will help you make wise choices. The Environmental Working Group regularly revises this list which is available on their website — www.ewg.org. The current listings are found below.

The Dirty Dozen		*The Cleanest*	
The 12 vegetables and fruit with the highest pesticide contamination. You may want to buy organic versions of these.		The 12 vegetables and fruit with the lowest pesticide contamination. The full list is found atwww.foodnews.org/fulllist.php	
Peach	Apple	Onion	Avocado
Bell Pepper	Celery	Frozen sweet corn	Pineapple
Nectarine	Strawberries	Mango	Asparagus
Cherries	Kale	Frozen sweet peas	Kiwi
Lettuce	Grapes (Imported)	Cabbage	Eggplant
Carrot	Pear	Papaya	Watermelon

You may also want to buy produce from local growers at farmer's markets. You can ask the grower if they use pesticides. Often they don't, even if they are not selling "certified" organic vegetables or fruit. Washing before eating can help remove pesticide residues on some vegetables and fruit. It also helps remove bacteria and other microbes. Always wash produce before you cut it up. There are some good vegetable wash solutions you can buy. You can also use the simple technique of adding one teaspoon mild soap in one gallon of water. Submerge produce in this soapy water and rinse well.

Consider these guidelines as well:
Use a vegetable brush on hard produce whose skin you plan to eat.
Peel wax- coated non-organic produce.
Discard outer leaves of lettuce and cabbage.

Protein-rich foods

A quick look at the Prudent diet and the Mediterranean diet shows a clear difference in protein sources from the Western diet. Less healthy choices include red meat, processed meats and high fat dairy foods. Healthier choices include chicken, low-fat dairy, and the best of all — fish and legumes.

You'll recall that we encourage you to follow some rules for eating. Some of you may decide to focus solely on plant protein sources. Others of you will choose to completely avoid red meat. And finally, most of you will choose healthier protein sources most of the time. But occasionally eat from the other list. If you want to stick exclusively to one approach, it works for us.

Protein-rich foods:
Eggs and egg whites
Fish
Chicken
Milk
Yogurt
Low fat cheese
Tofu
Edamame
Nuts and nut butter

Fish and legumes are considered the healthiest choices because of the nutrient contributions they make. In addition to providing protein, fish has omega-3 fatty acids that are protective against many diseases and inflammation in the body. Some species are higher in these healthy fats than others. Salmon, sardines, trout and mackerel are the richest sources. Choose fish carefully, though, because some species are contaminated with mercury. Others are in danger of being over fished, depleting their populations. A good resource for choosing fish comes from Seafood Watch and can be found on the Monterey Bay Aquarium website www.montereybayaquarium.org

Legumes or beans and dried peas are rich sources of soluble fiber, magnesium and folic acid, in addition to protein. Some of you may have the time to cook beans from scratch, but if you don't, canned beans are a good alternative. Compare nutrition labeling to pick a brand lower in sodium.

Don't overlook soy foods. Technically, soy foods fall into the category of legumes because they are made from beans. The best choices are soybeans themselves, edamame (immature green soybeans), soy nuts, tofu, tempeh and soy beverages.

What about soy and breast cancer?

As you may know, soy foods contain substances called isoflavones that have the ability to bind to estrogen receptors and have been considered to mimic the activity of estrogen to some degree. In some animal studies, these isoflavones stimulate the growth of breast cancer cells. This research led to a concern about the safety of soy foods for women with breast cancer. To date, studies on women have not shown a similar effect.

Most doctors and nutritionists now believe that soy foods are safe for women with breast cancer.

Healthy fats and oils

Many people think that fats and oils are nutritional "bad guys". But there are some surprises when you look closely at the facts about fats and oils. Some types are absolutely essential for staying healthy.

The healthy fats are, in general, unsaturated. Unsaturated says something about their physical characteristics. They are liquid at room temperature and called oils. There are two general types of healthy unsaturated oils

The first is monounsaturated oil, preferably from a relatively unrefined source like extra virgin olive oil or expeller-pressed canola oil. The foods rich in healthy monounsaturated oils include avocado, nuts and olives. This should be the main type of fat in your diet for cooking, salad dressing and little high-fat extras.

The second type of healthy oil is omega-3, found in oily fish like salmon and sardines, flaxseed, and walnuts. It is also found in eggs laid by hens fed a high omega-3 diet and a variety of fortified foods to which it is added. Try to have some source of omega-3 oil every day. If your diet doesn't provide it, consider a supplement.

Should I eat a low fat-diet?

This is certainly not a bad idea, but we encourage you to not make a low fat diet your primary focus. When you eat more healthy foods like vegetables, fruit, fish and whole grains, you generally eat less unhealthy fats.

The Mediterranean diet pattern is actually fairly high in fat and definitely healthy. The secret is the types of fats included - monounsaturated and omega-3. Do concentrate on including these healthy fats in your diet on a regular basis.

It also pays to remember that fat is a concentrated source of calories. If you eat too many calories, you will gain weight. So choose your fats and oils wisely and watch portions of everything.

Whole grains

Whole grains are the latest nutritional darlings and with good reason. Our over consumption of white flour and other refined grains has done us little good. The whole grain versions of breads, cereals, rice and pastas are healthy additions to your pantry. Whole grains are always associated with better health, and people who choose whole grain foods regularly eat a better diet in general. It is mostly habit, so begin by finding whole grain versions of the foods you use regularly and make them a part of your life.

Eating for a healthy weight

Being overweight seems to make it harder to beat cancer. The world of nutrition research is sometimes slow and deliberate. We expect that studies will show this in the future, but as yet losing weight after a cancer diagnosis hasn't been shown to help a person beat the disease. But, exercising and eating a healthy diet have! Quite frankly, these are the two best strategies for losing weight anyway. They are much better than "going on a diet." They are more likely to result in real lifestyle change. They have also been shown to work to help a person beat cancer even if weight loss doesn't result.

We do know that weight loss can help protect you against many other diseases. So, if you want to boost the weight loss potential of Boot Camp and healthy eating, consider these suggestions:

Stop the habit

Giving up a regular habit of sugar-sweetened beverages including soda, sports drinks, teas and juice drinks, is no doubt one of the best strategies for losing a few pounds and keeping it off. Count real fruit juice as a fruit serving, but don't use it to quench your thirst.

Keep a food diary

We often are just not aware of when, what and how much we eat. A food diary can bring your eating pattern into your awareness. It is only then that you can begin to make conscious decisions about eating differently. Ask yourself where the bulk of your calories are coming from. Are there foods you could easily cut out?

The food diary, which doesn't have to be elaborate, also works as a good tool for self-monitoring. The National Weight Control Registry, which studies people who have been successful at permanent weight loss, has found that on-going attention to your patterns is essential to keeping weight off.

Pay attention to your portions

Often meat and starch take up most of the plate at mealtime. Changing this around can help you consume fewer calories. Instead have at least half your plate be vegetables. Make your portions of vegetables large. Let small to medium size portions of meat and starchy foods make up the rest.

Chapter Eleven: Call To Action

The beginning of a national program

In December 2008, I was asked to attend a conference at Miraval Resort called "Life beyond Cancer." I was so excited to be able to debut my program to over 150 cancer survivors and oncology nurses from all over the country. I knew and believed this program worked here in Tucson since I nurtured it for five years. I have seen the growth and impact it had on our community, but how would others feel? Visitors who knew nothing about it? That was always an underlying fear I had.

I eagerly planned my presentation of my classes, even taking a trip out to Miraval before the event to walk the grounds and to prepare for teaching my Boot Camp class. I was also fortunate enough to be given the opportunity to have a booth for the four-day retreat to promote my program. I couldn't wait for the weekend to arrive.

Since this was a program that participants from the retreat could sign up for in their spare time, I wasn't sure if they would choose this class over a spa service. Luckily, the spa services were spread out all day and night, so there was some creative scheduling they could do to take in everything. I knew there would be some local Boot Camp members attending. I politely requested that they attend my classes while they were there. This way I knew it would ensure the class being full.

At Miraval, classes were posted on a sign-up sheet indicating how many people are planning on taking them. Class size is limited. I figured, what the hell, I'll limit it to 25. That should be my biggest problem to have a waiting list. To my surprise, not only did my regulars sign up, but others! I did notice that some signed up for multiple classes. I quickly realized that these folks wanted more than a taste of Boot Camp. One of those participants was Lynn.

Classes were usually held late afternoon, before dinner. Many of us would end up all going to dinner afterwards. We quickly became known as the "loud fun" group, and one that many people wanted to be with. On the second day, many people were taking pictures of us. Again, I noticed one person who did that was Lynn.

Lynn, a cancer survivor soon realized that this was a program she wanted to bring back to Ohio. She was at that time teaching a fitness class at her hometown YMCA. Lynn knows what she wants and doesn't stop until she gets it. She attended the classes and was a true believer.

The retreat at Miraval was a success to me, because I realized that out-of-town visitors could appreciate the program. I was satisfied.

In the past, there had been a few people who had an interest in starting this program elsewhere in the country, but I wasn't sure if they really had the drive to do it. I kept in contact with some. At this same time I was tying up loose ends with my attorney to license the program and protect it's integrity.

Lynn persisted in telling me she wanted to branch out with my Boot Camp program. She emailed me, sent me pictures of us together at the retreat to jog my memory of who she was. It didn't take me too long to understand that she would be the perfect person to help me achieve my goal of making this a national program.

We discussed this project for months, going over all the details. I felt very confident if anyone could do it and make it a success, Lynn could.

We finally came to an agreement, and I sent her the licensing contract. It didn't take her long to secure a grant from a health foundation. She began partnering with her local YMCA, with whom she already had a relationship. She met with oncologists and community leaders. She followed my guidance of setting up a foundation of support for the program.

Before I knew it, I was making reservations to fly out to Ohio for the kickoff! How exciting! I really didn't know what to expect. Suzanne, who was instrumental in helping me make the arrangements to take this program national, agreed to go with me. Her background was programming for spas and resorts. It was great to have her there to validate the program expansion firsthand.

To my delight, the weekend was a bigger success than I imagined. It started with my meeting the instructors for the classes and working with them. I had the pleasure of going to the YMCA to meet Dave, the director who played an important role in all this. How touched was I when I saw a whole table of Boot Camp gear displayed for everyone to see! That evening there was a dinner for me to meet some of the volunteers of the program with a reception to follow of around 40 community movers and shakers who believe in this.

I could hardly sleep that night, waiting for the big official kickoff. Beat Cancer Boot Camp now is a national program! That morning I arrived at the park at the YMCA, and they were setting up the stage for the speakers. Booths were getting organized for all the vendors.

I began the morning by running a class for all who showed up! There were probably 45 people, some survivors, some family, friends and supporters. I have to admit, it was kind of weird to see, my t-shirts, my logos, all over this Ohio town!

The workout was a blast. They loved it! I was thrilled. Soon after the class the kickoff began. There were many speakers; oncologists, the head of the foundation, and survivors, who all spoke on behalf of this program. I was so moved by the impact this was having so quickly and all the people who truly believed in it. There was even a proclamation from the Mayor proclaiming September 12, 2009, as "Beat Cancer Boot Camp" day.

Later that day, while I was sitting around talking with Lynn and Suzanne, Lynn asked why I picked her to be the first one to start this program. Truthfully there were others, but none that I felt had the heart and soul of the program that Lynn did. I told her the truth, that she hounded me for months until I finally got it — that if she wanted this program so badly, there was no way she was going to let it fail.

Lynn has graciously offered to talk to others interested in starting this program and will teach them the tricks of the trade, from grant writing, to building relationships in the community, to finding just the right instructors, and partnering with a local YMCA or park district. Her persistence paid off, not only for her city but for Boot Camp as well. We are now on our way to reaching out to people all over the country. I can't wait!

Doing this program for almost six years, I have seen it work. I have seen what a difference it makes to so many people, survivors and buddies as well. It is one of the most rewarding programs to be part of, and it's not fair to restrict this program to only my community. Cancer has touched so many people across the country, so why not let everyone benefit from Beat Cancer Boot Camp?

We have a licensed, registered program designed to help survivors and their buddies become physically stronger and, in turn, mentally tougher. The program has enabled many participants to conquer the obstacles that come their way, no matter what stage of treatment or recovery they are in. Exercise has been shown not only to prevent some cancers but to work against recurrence. This is a positive take-charge physical support group open to all. My goal is to reach out to all communities to help them start this program.

Visit the website at www.beatcancerbootcamp.com. Or email me at beatcancerbootcampinfo.com. I would be delighted to help you get this program to your community.

In 2008, I attended the "Life Beyond Cancer Retreat" at Miraval Resort in Tucson, Arizona, and learned a tremendous amount about many things, especially the importance of growth towards a new concept of wellness. I was also introduced to the energy that is Beat Cancer Boot Camp. I was in shock the first time I saw their spirit. I was peacefully eating breakfast and saw these crazy women at 7:00 am, running by in camouflage pants chanting "I don't care what you've been told, we are brave and we are bold . . ." My heart did a little flop and I joined in with Anita's class the next two mornings.

As a past fitness and spinning teacher, I knew that exercise, nutrition, and support groups are a must for cancer survivors. Studies have shown over and over again the correlation between reoccurrence of cancer and being physically and mentally healthy. Strength in Motion (SIM), a local exercise program for breast cancer survivors, had a waiting list for attendance this past year in my hometown. It was drawing in people from 4 adjoining counties. SIM was only for breast cancer patients due to the fact that it was partially funded by Susan G. Komen Grant funds. As the volunteer Project Director, it tore my heart out to turn away women with cervical, colon, lung and other types of cancers.

After a chat with Dave Tener, the CEO of our local YMCA, we decided to bring BCBC to Ohio. We wrote a grant to offset the initial costs to begin the program. The grant was approved and I formalized the agreement with the YMCA in the spring of 2009. We both felt very strongly that this new program is not OUR program, but is a community program.

The next step was to sell the merits of the program to the rest of the community, so Dave and I went to various organizations and explained to them what an awesome opportunity this was for our area to be able of offer a program for cancer survivors that would soon be highly recognized nationally. At about that time, Anita was featured in an article of Cure magazine, talking about fitness and fatigue, and we were able to leverage off of that piece.

After getting to know Anita, I understood her dream to have this program become recognized nationally. I know absolutely and without any reservation that Anita will insure that every spin-off will adhere to her high standards and that the integrity of the program will be preserved. Because of the direct correlation between health and cancer recurrence, BCBC is the perfect venue for survivors — offering exercise and a healthy support group atmosphere.

- Lynn B.

Several years ago, Pima County dedicated a portion of its award-winning Brandi Fenton Memorial Park in Tucson, Arizona for the first Beat Cancer Boot Camp site.

Instead of locating the wellness course and training site in some remote corner of the park, the course was designed and constructed along the park's most visible exposure along one of the county's most heavily traveled roads. Our goal was, and continues to be, to showcase and promote the program's participants, the facility and the positive outcomes that such bring.

This important program and creative partnership is increasingly receiving national recognition, some of which may be attributed to the innovative and cost effectiveness processes that it implements. In our case, Beat Cancer Boot Camp has provided the programming and related personnel; the county has provided the real estate and facilities. Thus, program and cost efficacy are maximized.

In 2007, the Beat Cancer Boot Camp program became the recipient of Pima County's "Most Outstanding Program" award. In fact, the county has seen such great success and demand for this program that it will soon be available county-wide at numerous parks. This will provide ease of access and participation to the region's residents.

There is no reason to wait in incorporating this program into the fabric of our communities. The social and economic implications are huge. As research has shown, there is a correlation on health and the economy. More importantly, there is a direct correlation between health and our personal and social well-being. Each and every day that we wait we miss the opportunity to reach out to help someone who is seeking hope. We are in the position of helping one another — unless we poorly chose to do otherwise.

- Rafael Payan,
Director of Pima County Natural Resources,
Parks and Recreation

Chapter Twelve: Reflections on Boot Camp

What drew me to Boot Camp? Two very important goals — to strengthen my body and my soul. One of my oncologists told me that the single most important thing I can do to reduce the risk of recurrence is to exercise, exercise, exercise. The other important part of Boot Camp is the camaraderie. All of us really care about and care for one another.

–Karen O.

When I finally got the courage to contact Sarge, she challenged be to join up by saying she'd seen "recruits" far older and in worse situations than mine do well in Boot Camp. Who were these women who had cancer but were brave enough to take a military style workout, outdoors in all kinds of weather? I had to see for myself.

Boot Camp turned out to be the best treatment of all. The workout itself is strenuous and rewarding, but Boot Camp offers even more. I've become part of a diverse group of women. Cancer survivors and buddies who are united by the common bond of having our lives touched by cancer, all wanting to take action and get stronger.

–Sarah S.

While going through chemotherapy, my white blood count became very low, making me susceptible to infection which, for a cancer patient, can be life threatening. As a physician, I had seen people die, not just from their cancer but from the complications of their treatments.

I became acutely aware of crowded places filled with people coughing and sneezing, and all the things they touched! A gym had become out of the question.

Having been made to feel at home at the Boot Camp lunches, I decided to try the exercise group. I was pretty weak and fatigued and still getting chemo, so I wasn't sure how it would go. Anita, our Sarge, made it clear to push ourselves but know our limitations. Just do what you can.

It felt great to be outdoors, away from the germs of the gym and in the company of really fun, encouraging women. Over the next several months, I began using heavier weights and noticed my body starting to regain its former strength and shape! I had more energy and was sleeping better at night.

–Liz A.

"I hate to exercise!" I told Liz every time she brought up Boot Camp. As a physician colleague and good friend, she told me how much she enjoyed this Boot Camp class, which was dedicated to people who had had cancer. Beat Cancer Boot Camp. She knew that I was not just her doctor buddy but also that I had had colorectal cancer diagnosed in 2000 with a couple of recurrences since then.

Liz and I had both gone through long rounds of chemo and radiation and I had experienced several pelvic surgeries that took months of recovery. The idea of heavy-duty exercise twice a week just did not sound that appealing, especially the push-ups! Yes, yes, yes, I knew of the data that indicated exercise helped to prevent recurrence and that consistent workouts are disease preventers — after all I am a doctor.

I will never forget the first two or three workouts. Because of my genera tenacity, I wanted to do everything that Sarge told us to do. Never mind that my thighs were screaming and I was panting at the end of each of the leg riffs. And I never knew that five pounds was so heavy! It was the repetitions that seemed ruthless. As we entered the Circle of Doom, as some of the others not so jokingly called the area of the park where we do pushups, I was just about done. But — I liked it! Even though I could barely lower myself to a chair the next few days, I was proud of myself. So, I kept going back. And back, and back.

What could be better than that?

–Lana H.

I never was thrilled about exercise, but once I saw the teamwork that was taking place, I too wanted to be part of this program. Yes, there still are days when I don't feel like going to Boot Camp, but knowing that my buddy and all my friends will be there helps me know that I will be benefiting myself through exercise.

–Ginny S.

I am a Boot Camp neophyte actively undergoing chemotherapy. Originally, a breast cancer support group was recommended to me by one of the local hospitals. However, when I attended my first session, I left feeling very depressed. The group dynamics were negative and provided all the unpleasant details of mastectomy, chemo, radiation and reconstruction issues. The women were nice, but I realized that the group wouldn't meet my needs, or my personality. Then I went to boot camp. I brought my son as my buddy and even he had fun and got a good workout. The women were varied in age, personality and cancer history and very open about their experiences if I asked. I left the session feeling energized and lucky to have found this group.

-Annie O.

Anita welcomed me to the Beat Cancer Boot Camp when I had no hair or eyelashes, and could barely hold a pencil from being so weak. She never looked at my physical appearance, but encouraged my spirit. I remember her coaxing me to lift weights and endure one more pushup.

Every workout I became a little bit stronger, and formed a bond with other survivors and supporters. Through these workouts a wonderful support group emerged, helping the community as well as each other with our individual lives.
–Brenda S.

Boot Camp is not the traditional support group. I found myself attracted to Anita's attitude, and it permeates all Boot Camp activities. The attitude here is we're strong, bold and fearless and we will fight with all our might. We exercise together with the goal that as we get stronger physically, we will get stronger emotionally and spiritually. We will do better than just survive cancer … we will THRIVE as survivors!
–Loretta H.

Cancer is a terrible thing. But it also has brought me blessings. Boot Camp is one of them! Not only the exercise, but also mostly the support of the women. When I need help getting to doctors appointments after surgery, I know I can ask for help from the group. I have made some wonderful new friendships and I am most grateful for these wonderful women!
–Arlene K.

Boot Camp is not about easy. It is about learning that we can do things that are hard. We can do things that are hard and thrive. Of course, hearing the diagnosis of cancer is devastating. Yet from the moment I heard it, I began a journey that, in retrospect, is truly one of the most positive experiences of my life. Boot Camp clearly teaches irony!

I learned to laugh loud and hard with others about our shapes, our challenges, our shared humanity. I learned to love and forgive others and myself, too. I learned to love others who do not necessarily agree with me on some issues, but whom I trust, respect, and admire.
–Celia P.

Originally, I joined the group to get in shape and to support my sister-in-law. Before I knew it, I was hooked! When you are at the 90th push up and ready to give up, you look over at these survivors and know you have to hang with them! Not only was I getting in shape, but I was helping make a difference in my life and the lives of those around me. In addition, I became a person who was part of a group that helped the community in a big way. Now THAT was important to me.

I have always been a positive person, but this group helped me appreciate every moment of my life

—Virginia E.

Cancer is a disease that you carry with you, no matter how long you've been in remission. Fear of recurrence can at times be paralyzing. Working out twice a week and seeing the many faces of the women of Boot Camp, helped keep those fears in check. I also knew that if I got in trouble again, I had many arms to support me.

—Rosanne H.

Well, let me tell you this group is far from traditional. I have never in my life, and I am 58 years old, met a group of women so outstanding, so vivacious, so positive, so energetic and so caring. The camaraderie within Boot Camp is amazing.

We drag ourselves to exercise. We complain while being there, but love it when we're through. Our muscles and bodies feel great. Everyone exercises at their own pace and within their comfort level. Such a proud feeling overcomes me whenever I am with this amazing group of women.

Besides the grueling exercising, we have incorporated a mentoring group, which i am proud to say I am involved with. We dine together, travel together, and depend on each other like sisters — this is our sisterhood. Thanks to Sarge, many lives are enriched, including mine. Beat Cancer Boot Camp rocks!

—Pam C.

When you are working out with all of these women, it is spiritual, there is a deep connection, and it is full of positive energy & strength. I look forward to the time that we spend together on a weekly basis. I wish that everyone who is going through cancer would have such an incredible support group. It is simply beyond anything that words could even begin to express!

—Tami B.

Although I had outstanding support from family and friends, I still felt so alone sometimes. Life is going on around you and yours has come to a screeching halt. You begin to wonder if you will ever have a normal life again. Boot Camp makes me feel like in many ways it's better than ever. It gives those of us who are new survivors such hope to be around women that have been surviving for many years.

The funny thing is when I recently went through my reconstructive surgery, I couldn't wait for the doctor to tell me I could get back to exercising so that I could return to Boot Camp. I really do miss it when I take any time off. I miss the workout, but most of all I miss my Boot Camp buddies.

–Pam J.

When my wife, Pam, was diagnosed with breast cancer in the fall of 2006, the news was a shock to our family.

The treatments ended and she was a survivor … but now what? The treatment battle was over but how would we know if she won the war? This is one of the heaviest of burdens to bear and there is no medicine for it.

Then Beat Cancer Boot Camp entered the picture. One of our daughters saw an article about the group and passed it along to Pam. One visit and she was hooked. Here were a bunch of women like her, in the same situation, and they were doing something about it. They were staying strong through physical exercise. They had positive attitudes. They supported one another. They were all hell-bent on survival. "Pity parties," as Pam calls them, were not allowed.

This new group of friends, in my view, gave Pam what was missing at the end of her treatment, a way to continue to fight the battle on her terms. The only difference? Now she has an entire army at her side fighting with her.

–Mike J.

Three weeks before my wedding, I was told I had breast cancer. My first concern was whether I would survive.

When Anita first told me about BCBC I wasn't that enthusiastic about attending. I'm not a very social person and wasn't interested in a "crying" support group. However I found that it is not only a good group to get a great workout, but I can talk about problems I'm having with or as a result of my treatment. This is the perfect because I can ask questions of the other survivors for tips on handling issues. Believe me, when you go through your treatment, whether it's surgery, chemotherapy, radiation or all three you'll have problems. This is not the time to be shy about discussing them so having this network of women survivors has been a godsend. I'm so thankful Anita founded this group; it's been good for me physically and mentally.

–Kathy L.

The physical challenge part is not what has kept me going to Boot Camp for the last five or so years. I keep going to Beat Cancer Boot Camp because it's the only place where I have been able to take control of a small but significant portion of my newly acquired sense of mortality. I am challenged and motivated every week in Boot Camp to take good physical care of this life and to expand that goodness to improve my mental and emotional health too.

–Nancy P.

Being diagnosed with breast cancer thrust me into a club I had no interest in joining. Being identified as a sick person made no sense in my conscientious, healthy lifestyle. I felt my spirit draining of its strength and optimism. I couldn't remember the tools I normally use when life would get turned upside down. Fear and anger just cried itself out of me threatening to drown me out of my very existence.

At boot camp, women share their hearts through their stories and the flashing of scars and beautiful newly reconstructed breasts. They opened their hearts and this made it safe and welcoming for me to open mine. It is healing. It is connection. It is community.

–Shawn M.

I initially joined up with Beat Cancer Boot Camp for the fitness and the belief that I had so much to give. At first I almost felt guilty because I was a "buddy" and not a "survivor," but like most people my life has been changed by cancer in one way or another.

We all play a part and are vital to the team experience. What a brilliant concept. Bring a diverse group of women together to fight one common fight — cancer. To laugh, cry, support, encourage and inform. They take an interest in everyone's personal story and take that story to the public to increase awareness and promote good health.

These ladies have changed my life with their courage, humor, compassion and desire to live the best life possible. Their passion and vitality is contagious to those around them.

-Margo S.

I have been going to Boot Camp almost 4 years now, and while it soon became clear to me how much I was getting out of the exercise program, much more slowly I discovered how important the support group component of Beat Cancer Boot Camp is to me.

I now feel Boot Camp is kind of my home away from home. I think because we share a common bond and we open up to each other sharing our trials and tribulations of the various treatments we are going through, a special closeness develops that lets genuine friendships grow. Whether it's waiting for results from a new biopsy or dealing with personal issues totally unrelated to my health, my boot camp buddies are there for me, offering me support, hope, and love. And to each of them, I say thank you.

-Dawn M.

I joined Boot Camp to find something to give back to the community that was different than I had ever done before. When I first began I thought to myself ... what am I doing, I'm sixty years old.

I saw all the survivors exercising and here I was huffing and puffing. But I kept coming back. These women were my inspiration and role models.

-Marlyne F.

At 29, I was diagnosed with hypertension. Being 60 years old, I have been fighting this disease for many years. I progressively took more pills to maintain my blood pressure and I dreaded having to rely on medication to remain healthy.

Though I didn't have cancer, I thought this would be something helpful for me and I joined right away. A couple months later after exercising, I felt faint. I immediately made an appointment with my doctor. To my surprise, I lost 10 pounds and my blood pressure had dropped. My medication has now been cut in half. This was a first.

-Linda S.

Afterword

This is a difficult thing for me to put in words. I've been asked this time and time again, what does Boot Camp mean to me? It would be too simple to answer in one word. EVERYTHING.

I have put my heart and soul into this for several years. It takes up countless hours of the day. It is always on my mind. It is all consuming. Would I have it any other way? I don't know how. This program is so important to me, because it is important to so many others. It has made a difference in lives, and that's what keeps me going.

Sometimes, I'll just chuckle to myself thinking of something funny that happened that day at class. They constantly crack me up. Some days I hold back the tears, knowing what they are going through that particular moment. It is sometimes difficult to keep their spirits up, but I try. All they need is support and security of knowing they are not alone. That's what this program does. How quickly the importance of this group becomes to all of us.

Two years ago, as I was approaching my 50th birthday, I knew my husband was probably planning a big surprise party for me. All I had to do was figure out a sneaky way to take a peek at the guest list. Yep, I was right. He was planning a party to celebrate my big birthday. The problem was, he had no idea who my real friends were, who I felt closest with. I knew he would go through all my old guest lists from previous parties and invite everyone, thinking they would all like to be part of this.

The people I felt closest with, the ones I want to celebrate milestones with, were my troops from Boot Camp. Knowing there was no tactful way to approach this, I dealt with this head on like I know best. I came straight out and asked him, hoping it wouldn't hurt his feelings by taking out the surprise element out of this day. It was more important to me, to be surrounded by family and friends, who are there for me as I am to them.

I was thankful he was quick to understand and change the party list. It meant the world to me to be able to celebrate my special day with people that matter and make a difference in my life. As much as they praise me for what I've done for them, it is nothing in return for what they have done for me.

I have to tell you I was quite taken aback when the troops gave a performance at my party. The fact that they were secretly rehearsing this behind my back caught me off guard. The little skit they performed, along with some personalized cadences designed for this event were hilarious.

For example, here was my special birthday song:

Sarge is tough, we know too well,
Stick with her your muscles swell,
We all moan, she says don't whine,
Or you'll do it double time.

She'll dial your number, don't you ditch.
It's cause she cares, but she's a bit … nice person!
She makes us work out, cold and rain,
We pay for this, it's just insane.

But still you're here, you keep us strong
Deep down we've loved you all along.
So thank you, Sarge, you are the best.
You're short but stand above the rest!

It was a great birthday, celebrating with my family and troops! I am so glad I spoke up and didn't wait for my husband to try to pull off a big surprise party without the people I really wanted to spend time with!

For Strength. For Health. For Life.
–Anita